Viva la Vulva

Dr. Christopher Jenner

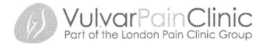

Viva la Vulva

Viva la Vulva, London, United Kingdom

Website: www.vulvarpainclinic.com

PR Enquiries: **info@vulvarpainclinic.com**

ISBN: 978-1-7399091-1-6 (paperback)

A CIP catalog record for this book is available from the British Library.

Editors

Dr. Ingrid Bergson, PsychD. (Hons)
Consultant Clinical Psychologist
London Orthopedic Clinic and London Bridge Hospital
HCA
London, UK

Dr. Arun Bhaskar, MBBS, MSc, FRCA, FFPMRCA, FFICM, FIPP
Consultant in Pain Medicine
Imperial Healthcare NHS Trust
London, UK

Dr. Micheline Byrne, MB, BCh, MRCOG, BAO
Consultant in Genitourinary Medicine and Vulvologist
Honorary Senior Lecturer
Imperial Healthcare NHS Trust
London, UK

Professor Linda Cardoza, OBE, MD, FRCOG
Professor of Urogynaecology
Consultant Gynecologist
Department of Urogynecology
King's College Hospital
London, UK

Ms. Jennifer Constable, MCSP, AACP, MPOGP
Consultant Pelvic Health Physiotherapist
Six Physio
London, UK

Dr. Mike Cummings, MB, ChB, Dip Med Ac
Medical Director
British Medical Acupuncture Society
Royal London Hospital for Integrated Medicine
London, UK

Dr. Jose De Andres, MD, PhD, FIPP, EDRA, EDPM

Past President European Society of Regional Anesthesia and Pain Therapy (ESRA)
Vice Chairman European Diploma of Pain Medicine (EDPM-ESRA)
Tenured Professor of Anesthesia. Valencia School of Medicine
Chairman Anesthesia Critical Care and Pain Management Department
General University Hospital
Avda Tres Cruces s/n.46014 Valencia. Spain.

Dr. Alex Digesu, MD, PhD

Consultant in Obstetrics & Gynecology
Urogynaecology Subspecialist
Imperial College Healthcare NHS Trust
London, UK

Dr. Robert J. Echenberg, MD, FACOG

Specialist in Pelvic, Genital and Sexual Pain
Lecturer, Author and Clinician
The Echenberg Institute
Pennsylvania, US

Maria Elliott, BSc (Hons), MCSP, HCPC

Pelvic Health Physiotherapist
CEO and Founder of Mummy MOT
Maria Elliott Physiotherapy Services
4 Upper Wimpole Street
London, UK

Dr. Gustavo Fabregat-Cid, MD, PhD, FIPP, EDPM

Consultant in Pain Medicine
University General Hospital, Valencia
Associate Professor
Catholic University, Valencia, Spain

Dr. Charles A. Gauci, OLM, KCHS, MD, FRCA, FIPP, FFPMRCA, RAMC (Retd)

Former Consultant in Pain Medicine, Whipps Cross University
    Hospital
London, UK
Former Hon. Consultant in Pain Medicine, Guy's & St. Thomas'
    Hospital
London, UK
Consultant in Pain Medicine
Mater Dei Hospital
Malta

Dr. Lorraine Sarah Harrington, MBChB, Bsc (Hons), MRCP, FRCA, FFPMRCA

Consultant in Pain Medicine
NHS Lothian
Edinburgh, UK

Miss Anne Henderson, MA, MBBChir, MRCOG

Consultant Gynecologist
Owner and Clinical Director
The Amara Clinic
2 Linden Close
Tunbridge Wells
Kent, UK

Dr. Christopher Arthur Jenner, MB BS, FRCA, FFPMRCA

Consultant in Pain Medicine
Honorary Clinical Lecturer
Imperial Healthcare NHS Trust
London, UK

Mr. Nathaniel S. Jones, Jr., BS, R.Ph., FAPC

Clinical Compounding Pharmacist
Professional Compounding Centers of America
Houston, Texas, US

Professor Vikram Khullar, BSc, MB BS, MRCOG, MD, AKC

Consultant in Obstetrics & Gynecology
Urogynaecology Subspecialist
Imperial College Healthcare NHS Trust
London, UK

Ms Marta Kinsella, BSc (Hons), HCPC, MCSP, PGOP
Pelvic Health and Rehabilitation Physiotherapist
Beyond Health
Parsons Green
London, UK

Dr. Susan Kellogg Spadt, PhD, CRNP, IF, FCST
Director of Female Sexual Medicine
Center for Pelvic Medicine
Bryn Mawr, Pennsylvania, US
Prof OBGYN at Drexel University College of Medicine
Philadelphia, Pennsylvania, US

Dr. Kim Lawson, BTech (Hons), PhD
Senior Lecturer in Pharmacology
Sheffield Hallam University
Sheffield, UK

Dr. Yi Liu, PharmD, PhD, R.Ph
Research Pharmacist
Research & Development Department
Professional Compounding Centers of America
Houston, Texas, US

Dr. Deirdre Lyons, MB BCh, BAO, MRCOG
Consultant in Gynecology
St. Mary's Hospital
Imperial Healthcare NHS Trust
London, UK

**Dr. Jawaad Saleem Malik, BSc (Hons), MB BS, Executive
   MBA, MFMLM, MAcadMEd, FRCA**
Specialist Registrar in Pain Medicine
Advanced Pain Fellow
Imperial Healthcare NHS Trust
London, UK

Dr. Pamela Morrison Wiles, PT, MS, DPT, BCB-PMD, IMTC
Pelvic Pain Expert, Author, Speaker
Pamela Morrison Physical Therapy, PC
140 West End Ave., Suite 1K
New York, N.Y. 10023, US

Professor Filippo Murina, MD

Professor and Chief
Lower Genital Tract Disease Unit
Obstetrics and Gynecology Department
V. Buzzi Hospital
University of Milan
Milan, Italy

Dr. Sunny Nayee, MB BChir (Cantab), FRCA, FFPMRCA

Consultant in Pain Medicine
Imperial Healthcare NHS Trust
London, UK

Dr. John Newbury-Helps, DClinPsych, MA, MBA

Specialist Clinical Psychologist
Imperial Healthcare NHS Trust
London, UK

Mr. Angus McIndoe, PhD, FRCS, MRCOG

Consultant Gynecologist
The McIndoe Centre
9 Harley Street
London, UK

Miss Anusha Patel, MPharm (Hons)

Head Pharmacist
Pharmacierge
Wimpole Street
London, UK

Dr. Anna Pallecaros, MB BS, MRCP, BSc, DSTD, DTM&H, DFSRH

Consultant in Genitourinary Medicine & Sexual Health
The Harley Street Clinic Diagnostic Centre
HCA Healthcare
London, UK

Dr. Michael Platt, MA, MB BS, FRCA, FFPMRCA

Consultant in Pain Medicine
Honorary Clinical Lecturer
Imperial Healthcare NHS Trust
London, UK

Dr. Ivan Nin Ramos-Galvez, LMS, FRCA, FFPMRCA
Consultant in Pain Medicine
Royal Berkshire NHS Foundation Trust
Reading, UK

Dr. Attam Singh, MB BS, FRCA, FFPMRCA
Consultant in Pain Medicine
West Hertfordshire Hospitals NHS Trust,
Hertfordshire, UK

Dr. Amy Stenson, MD, MPH
Associate Professor
Residency Program Director
Oregon Health & Science University
Portland, Oregon, US
Department of Obstetrics and Gynecology
3181 SW Sam Jackson Drive
Portland, Oregon, US

Miss Petra Rosario, MPharm (Hons)
Pharmacist
Pharmacierge
Wimpole Street
London, UK

Ms. Riikka Uljas-Bärman, MA
Organization Coordinator
The Gynecological Patient Association Korento ry
Finland
Community Educator
Finland

Mr. Edward Ungar, MA (Cantab), MBA
CEO Pharmacierge
Pharmacierge
Wimpole Street
London, UK

Mr. Leon Ungar, MRPharmS
Co-Founder and Pharmacist Director
Pharmacierge
Wimpole Street
London, UK

Ms. Sarah Wolujewicz, BSc (Hons), Postgrad Cert, HCPC, MCSP, MPOGP

Clinical Lead, Pelvic Health Physiotherapy
Imperial College Healthcare NHS Trust
London, UK
Pelvic Health Physiotherapist
The Havelock Clinic
London, UK

Disclaimer

Although the author and publisher have made every effort to ensure that the information in this book is correct at the time of publication, the author and publisher do not assume and hereby disclaim any liability to any party for any loss, damage, or disruption caused by errors or omissions, whether such errors or omissions result from negligence, accident, or any other cause.

This book is not intended as a substitute for the medical advice of physicians. The reader should regularly consult a physician in matters relating to their health, particularly with respect to any symptoms that may require diagnosis or medical attention.

The information contained in the e-book, paperback, hardback, and audiobook (together referred to as 'Material'), is for general information purposes, and nothing contained in it is, or is intended to be, construed as advice, unless the suggestion/s have been approved by the reader's personal physician or personal healthcare provider. This is because it does not consider the reader's individual health, medical, physical, or emotional situation or needs. It is not a substitute for medical attention, treatment, examination, advice, treatment of existing conditions or diagnosis, and is not intended to provide a clinical diagnosis, nor take the place of proper medical advice from a fully qualified medical practitioner.

Prior to acting on, or using any of the information herein, the reader/listener must consider its appropriateness regarding their own personal situation and requirements. Readers/listeners are responsible for consulting a suitable medical professional prior to trying out any treatment or taking any course of action that may directly or indirectly affect their physical or mental health or wellbeing, because of what they have read or heard in the Material.

To the maximum extent permitted by law, the author and publisher disclaim all responsibility and liability to any person, arising directly or indirectly from any person acting or not acting based on the information in the Material.

Introduction

Smashing the Stigma

Up to 16% of women experience vulvodynia at some point in their lives, regardless of age, ethnicity, or socioeconomic group. The pain of vulvodynia can upend relationships and turn daily life into a nightmare. Then there is the stigma that vulvodynia carries. Many women are embarrassed to discuss vulvar pain with their doctors, and the taboo on women's health topics doesn't help. A lack of open discussion means that thousands of women worldwide are suffering in silence with no hope of a cure.

But the idea that you have to suffer in silence is a lie. There are plenty of ways to treat vulvodynia, and with help, it's 100% possible to take back control of your life and relationships. In this book, we're going to smash the stigma and empower you with the knowledge you need to rid yourself of vulvar pain.

This book was written for you by practicing physicians, pelvic physiotherapists, and scientists with years of experience treating vulvodynia and vulvar pain in patients. Some of our patients suffered for years before getting help, and we know how hard it can be to break the stigma and ask for that help. That's why we put our brains together and wrote this book.

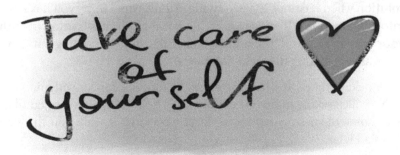

It's not a thesis or a physician's manual. It's an easy-to-read, step-by-step approach. We'll discuss available treatments for vulvodynia, self-help options, and guidance for everyday management—all in layman's terms with simple illustrations. At the end of each chapter, you'll find references that you can look up for more detailed information.

Hopefully, this book will help you work with your physician, pelvic physiotherapist, or other pelvic healthcare professional to get treatment. Think of it as your go-to guide to crushing vulvar pain.

Of course, there's no single magic bullet cure for vulvodynia, and we recognize that there are many potential treatments available. Not all patients respond to treatments in the same way. As with anything, there's always a certain amount of trial and error involved. That's why we recommend a whole-body approach with regular monitoring and check-ups, so you and your physician can gauge how well treatment is working for you.

As a Specialist Consultant in Pain Medicine at Imperial Healthcare NHS Trust, and as the Director of the London Pain Clinic in Harley Street, London, UK, I've been treating patients with vulvodynia for many years using this multidisciplinary approach.

Ultimately, the goal of treatment is to reduce vulvar pain and make healing possible. In helping my own patients with vulvodynia, I always start with simple steps. For example, I might prescribe oral and topical medication, physiotherapy, and pelvic floor exercises to be done at home. If these simple treatments don't make a difference, I'll talk to my patient about more involved options, like minimally invasive pain medicine procedures and surgical intervention.

The point is, every case is different, and there's no one-size-fits-all solution when it comes to vulvodynia. That's why I hope you'll use the information in this book as a starting point to discuss treatment with your physician. And remember, the first step to getting effective treatment is getting the right diagnosis.

Luckily, there are many treatment options for vulvodynia, and we've collected the main ones in the table below. If you're not familiar with some of these treatments, don't worry: we'll walk you through them all later.

Treatment Options for Vulvodynia

Category	Treatment Option
Medication	Oral Medication Topical Medication Medical Cannabis

Physical Therapy	Pelvic Floor and Muscle Rehabilitation
	  Exercises
	Biofeedback
	Desensitization using Dilators and
	  Vibrators
	Pelvic Floor Training Chairs

Minimally Invasive
  Pain Medicine
  Procedures
	Nerve Blocks
	Botox Treatment
	Radiofrequency Treatment

Advanced Pain Medicine Procedures	Sacral Neuromodulation
Diet	Foods and Supplements
Complementary and Alternative Medicine	Acupuncture Vaginal Acupressure Manual Trigger Point Therapy TENS Yoga and Diaphragmatic breathing
Psychology	CBT Mindfulness
Surgery	Surgical Intervention

Self Help	Relationships
	Sexual Intimacy
	Pregnancy and Giving Birth
	Research Trials
	Organizations, Online Health
	  Communities (OHC) and Support
	  Groups
	Disability Benefits

One final piece of advice before we get started. As you review the information in this book, please keep in mind the following facts about medical treatment for vulvodynia:

- It's not an exact science.
- It can be complicated.
- It may require some trial and error.
- It may take a little while to work.
- What ends up working will be different for everyone.
- The best approach combines multiple options.

Now, let's smash the stigma and work on helping you feel better one step at a time.

"An individualized, holistic, and often multidisciplinary approach is needed to effectively manage the patient's pain and pain-related distress" [7].

Dr. Christopher A. Jenner, MB BS, FRCA, FFPMRCA
Consultant in Pain Medicine
Honorary Clinical Lecturer
Imperial Healthcare NHS Trust
London, UK

A Patient's View

Ten years ago, I was in pain. I was 30, single, and watching all my married friends start to have babies. At that time, it seemed I was destined for a life of painful sex, or no sex at all. I was numb from a bad breakup, numb from doctors shrugging their shoulders at me, numb from just having to live with it. The pain was ruining my life—not just my sex life, but my whole life. Beyond the pain lay doubt, dashed future dreams, sadness, anger, resentment. An array of gynecologists were patronizing and unsympathetic. "Nothing's wrong with your anatomy," I was told, while anything that touched me down there cut and stung, burning like a ring of fire. One female doctor said to me, impatiently, "You need to relax for me. It doesn't hurt." Another stated, "Sex will get better, you just need practice. Have some wine."

If you are reading this, you are likely in the same boat I was in when I picked up a book about Vulvodynia in hopes that it would help me figure out what was "wrong with me." I recall trying to get through the pages of that book but being unable to. There was so much useful information, but I was emotionally distraught, and the medical terms were of little comfort. I want to reassure you of some things before you begin reading this book. There is a lot of information in these pages. Some of it will be helpful, some of it may not apply directly to your situation and so may seem overwhelming. Be steadfast and gentle with yourself as you digest the information and stories you will find here.

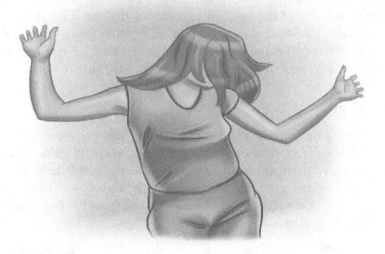

About 5 years ago, after sharing my story publicly, I started receiving notes from women all over the world. The notes came via Facebook, Instagram, and email. They came directly to me or were forwarded to me via the National Vulvodynia Association. If there had ever been a time when I felt I was alone, that feeling has long been dispersed as myth. One such note, from a 19-year-old woman, read, "I just want to feel that intimate, emotional connection with someone so desperately and I can't...how did you survive it and are you still ok now??"

I did survive it, and you can too. You need exactly three things to survive vulvodynia: a voice, a vocabulary, and your own volition.

Voice

Without a way of telling our story we are cut off from being able to heal. Carrying a secret is exhausting and makes a wound that will not heal until the matter is given words and witness. Take courage and find a way to confide in friends or loved ones who will truly listen. Many women have dealt with the same thing you are dealing with, and you will hear their voices in the pages of this book. Join them.

Vocabulary

The proper vocabulary will greatly aid your journey to wellness. It will be much easier to seek treatment and diagnosis when you have some knowledge of the medical approaches that have helped other women. Use the vocabulary you will find in these pages to pinpoint your symptoms and bolster your knowledge so that you are well equipped to discuss your condition with your medical provider.

Volition

Gather your courage and use all the force of your own will to seek and find the caring doctors who will listen to you and guide you on your journey. There are many incredibly knowledgeable helpers and healers for women suffering from vulvodynia, and if your doctor isn't one of them, take everything you have learned from the pages of this book and go find one who is.

A therapist said to me once, "Like driving at night, you have to keep moving to see what's ahead." Let this book, and the words of someone who has been in your shoes, give you some courage to keep going. To the friends, loved ones, and medical providers who are reading this book to educate themselves in support of a woman they know—thank you for being here. You are key to her healing process. Your love and support, and your willingness to hear her and to listen, are invaluable to the success of her journey.

Callista Jane Wilson
San Francisco, California, US
www.callistajanewilson.com

Callista is a former fashion stylist turned writer whose personal experiences with Vulvodynia led her to begin focusing on advocacy and awareness for women struggling with this devastating condition. She has been interviewed by the BBC Worldwide Radio, has had a play written and performed in London inspired by her story, and has published articles, written a book foreword, and produced a YouTube PSA sponsored by the National Vulvodynia Association. She gave birth to her first child, a son, in March 2019 and is currently working on her first book, a memoir. She lives in San Francisco, California, US.

A Doctor's View

Vulvodynia can have life-changing and negative impacts on women suffering from it. Not only is it a chronic pain condition, but it can also adversely affect day-to-day living, work, family life, and sexuality. As pain management services for women are fragmented, this book comes at a time where there is a clear need to provide a multidisciplinary approach to the problem.

Shortfalls in healthcare training and clinical interest have hitherto contributed to a widely held misperception that the condition is beyond treatment. As a result, many women have not had their diagnosis explained or their treatments optimized adequately. However, more recent medical research into the condition has exposed such misperceptions. A detailed history and clinical assessment alongside an understanding of the patient's individual needs can offer a variety of possible effective treatments. The delineation and exploration of such treatments is the central focus of this book.

A further challenge is to raise the awareness of both the healthcare workforce and the public to the intricacies of this condition. This should then enable more women to be seen by the correct health professionals. Early diagnosis, appropriate treatment, and self-management strategies will make a significant improvement to the lives of many.

This book is an essential contribution to our developing knowledge of this complex but widely prevalent and life-changing disease. Readers are provided with an excellent framework with which to help self-manage their condition. It will also serve as an essential resource for those health professionals working across all areas of women's health.

Dr. David Nunns, MD, FRCOG
Chair of the British Society for the Study of Vulval Disease
Trustee of the Vulval Pain Society
Consultant Gynecological Oncologist
Nottingham University Hospitals NHS Trust, UK

Table of Contents

Chapter 1

What is Vulvodynia?

"Vulvodynia is persistent, unexplained vulvar pain, which can affect women of all ages" [1].

Vulvar Pain

Most women will experience vulvar pain at some point in their lives. Based on how long it lasts, the pain is classified as either acute or chronic. Conditions that cause acute pain, which lasts less than three months, are usually easy to diagnose and manage. Chronic vulvar pain (CVP) is pain that lasts three months or more. There are many causes of chronic vulvar pain- some common, others rare. Diagnosing and managing CVP is more of a challenge. The commonest cause of CVP is a condition called vulvodynia, or VD.

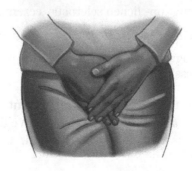

What is Vulvodynia?

Over the last 40 years, there has been some confusion about what vulvodynia actually is. In the seventies, it was used to describe burning vulvar pain. Sometimes, people used it to refer to any type of vulvar pain. The International Society for the Study of Vulvovaginal Disease (ISSVD) has worked very hard in recent years to clear up this confusion. Thanks largely to their efforts, vulvodynia is now a precise diagnosis. The ISSVD's current definition is:

"Chronic vulvar discomfort, most often described as burning pain, occurring in the absence of relevant visible findings or a specific, clinically identifiable, neurologic disorder."

Vulvodynia is a diagnosis of exclusion. In other words, when other possible causes of vulvar pain have been ruled out, doctors diagnose the condition as vulvodynia. The exact cause of vulvodynia is not known, but it is regarded as one of the most severe types of nerve or neuropathic pain. For doctors and clinicians, the ISSVD recommends the following classification to help diagnose women suffering from vulvar pain. First, clinicians should consider possible causes like infection, inflammation, neoplasia, and neurological conditions, as follows:

Vulvar pain related to a specific disorder – NOT vulvodynia

1. Infection- thrush, bacterial vaginosis etc.

2. Inflammation- lichen sclerosus, eczema etc.

3. Neoplasia- Paget's disease, carcinoma etc.

4. Neurological- pudendal nerve entrapment, spinal nerve compression etc.

If none of the above disorders are present, clinicians should consider vulvodynia, and classify it as follows. We'll look at what each of these classifications mean in the next section.

Vulvodynia

1. Generalized- multiple areas of the vulva affected
   a. Provoked- sexual, non-sexual, or both
   b. unprovoked
   c. mixed- both provoked and unprovoked
2. Localized- one area of the vulva affected
   a. Provoked- sexual, non-sexual, or both
   b. unprovoked
   c. mixed- both provoked and unprovoked

Obviously, it's vital for clinicians to correctly diagnose vulvodynia, and to be as specific as possible in their diagnosis. This will help women suffering from vulvodynia find relief more quickly and more completely.

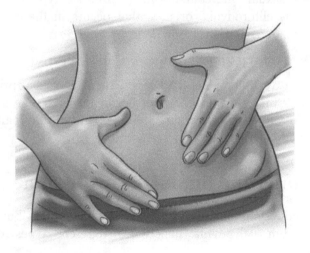

Subtypes of Vulvodynia

Generalized Vulvodynia

Generalized vulvodynia (GV) refers to pain in multiple areas of the vulva. The pain may fluctuate, with flares and remissions, and you may even experience some pain-free periods. Sexual intercourse usually aggravates the pain, as does sitting for long periods of time and performing other activities that put pressure on the vulva [4]. If you are diagnosed with generalized provoked vulvodynia, that means there's a clear trigger for the pain. But more often, generalized vulvodynia is unprovoked, meaning there's no clear trigger; the pain simply occurs spontaneously. Even so, certain activities, like intercourse, can still aggravate it.

Localized Vulvodynia

Women suffering from localized vulvodynia experience pain in only one part of the vulva. The most common type of vulvodynia is provoked localized vestibulodynia (PVD, previously called vulvar vestibulitis). Women with this condition experience burning, stinging, rawness, and irritation in the vulvar vestibule. Pressure on the tissues of the vestibule triggers this pain, usually caused by one or a combination of the following: foreplay, a gynecological examination, prolonged sitting, tampon insertion, wearing tight clothes, and penetrative sexual intercourse [4,12]. Another type of localized vulvodynia is clitorodynia, or pain that occurs in the clitoris, the genital organ in front of the vagina.

PVD: Primary and Secondary Classification

Provoked vestibulodynia (PVD), may be diagnosed as primary or secondary. Primary means the pain began the first time a woman experienced vaginal penetration. Secondary means the pain began after a period of pain-free vaginal penetration [4].

Symptoms and Signs of Vulvodynia

The main symptom of vulvodynia is vulvar pain, but women suffering from vulvodynia experience different types of pain, including:

- Pain over the inner vulva at the entrance to the vagina, especially during sex and when touched

- Uncomfortable burning and/or tingling sensations in the vulva

- Soreness, aching, and throbbing

- Pain and discomfort triggered by pressure to the tissues, such as from tight clothes and attempted tampon insertion [1,3,4,5,6]

Other symptoms include:

- Swelling

- Pain, frequency, or urgency with urination

When examining a patient for vulvodynia, clinicians may not see anything wrong other than some redness. As the patient, this can be very frustrating. You know there's something wrong because you're in intense pain, but the clinician may tell you they can't see anything. If this happens, you may want to ask your clinician to check for vulvodynia using other methods.

For example, since there are often no visual indicators of vulvodynia, clinicians may use the Pain Provocation Test, in which they use a light touch stimulus to test for pain. If pain occurs after a light touch that shouldn't normally cause pain (this reaction is known as allodynia), the patient may have vulvodynia. In other cases, clinicians may test for pain using a painful stimulus to see if the patient experiences more pain than is normal (this reaction is known as hyperalgesia).

Tenderness, tightness, and weakness of the pelvic floor muscles can also be signs of vulvodynia. 80% of vulvodynia sufferers experience pelvic floor muscle dysfunction.

Who Does Vulvodynia Affect?

Vulvodynia affects adolescents and adult women of all ages, ethnic backgrounds, races, and religions [6]. It is often linked to co-morbidities (other conditions), including recurrent cystitis, bladder pain syndrome, fibromyalgia, headache, endometriosis, constipation, irritable bowel syndrome, and other chronic pain conditions [6].

What Percentage of Women Suffer?

According to the National Vulvodynia Association, "Research studies find that as many as 16% of women in the US suffer from vulvodynia at some point in their lives. The highest incidence of symptom onset is between the ages of 18 and 25. The lowest incidence is after age 35" [6].

The Impact of Vulvodynia

For women suffering from vulvodynia, sexual intercourse is either impossible or painful. This can lead to women being embarrassed or afraid to start relationships [5]. In the worst cases, vulvodynia can lead to relationship issues, divorce, general sex problems, and sleep disturbances [6,10].

Some women are forced to leave their jobs because they can't sit at a desk. Others can't wear trousers or shorts, and some can't even wear underwear. Needless to say, these limitations often lead to feelings of hopelessness and depression, common among women with vulvodynia [6].

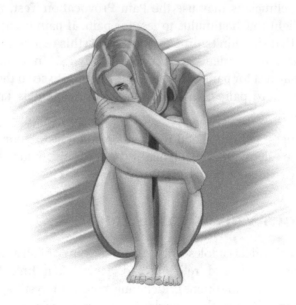

What Causes Vulvodynia?

While the exact cause of vulvodynia is not known, possible causes may include:

- Genetic susceptibility leading to overreaction/sensitivity to inflammation/infection

- Injury or irritation to the vulva nerves
- Changes in hormone levels
- Overreaction to injury/infection in the vulva cells
- Excess nerve fibers within the vulva
- Weakened pelvic floor muscles
- Allergic reaction to specific chemicals [10]

According to Harvard Health, "One theory is that it involves injury to the pudendal nerve, which runs from the lower spine to the vulva and vagina" [7]. This nerve damage could stem from a number of causes, including herpes zoster virus (the virus responsible for chickenpox and shingles), injury to the tail bone, a ruptured disc, childbirth, or pelvic surgery. Since the pudendal nerve is the principal nerve involved in vulvodynia, clinicians may target it when administering treatment [7].

Women who suffer from pain associated with intercourse, i.e., dyspareunia or vaginismus, often go on to develop vulvodynia, particularly if they experience vulvar pain before their first sexual experience or during their early experiences [8]. For some women, vulvodynia may also be connected to changes in estrogen levels, a history of urinary tract infections, HPV, and vaginal yeast infections. In fact, several researchers believe that repeated vaginal infections lead to long-term vulvodynia [7,9].

Common Misconceptions

Myth: STIs cause vulvodynia

STIs (sexually transmitted infections) do not cause vulvodynia [10]. This is a very common misconception that only contributes to the stigma around women's health. It's important to realize that if you suffer from vulvar pain or vulvodynia, it is not your fault. Practicing safe sex and getting vaccinated against STDs, while certainly beneficial to your overall health, will not help prevent vulvodynia.

Myth: Vulvodynia increases your cancer risk

There's a myth that having vulvodynia increases your risk of contracting cancer. This is simply not true. However, some types of cancer can cause pain in the vulvar region and may feel very similar to vulvodynia symptoms [8]. That's simply another reason to get any vulvar pain checked out by a specialist.

Myth: Vulvodynia is "all in your mind"

In the past, many women were told that vulvar pain was simply psychological. Fortunately, more healthcare professionals today are realizing that vulvodynia is a valid condition many women suffer from. And there's plenty of evidence now that vulvar pain can exist whether or not someone also suffers from anxiety, depression, or other mental and emotional health disorders. In other words, women who suffer from vulvodynia are not simply laboring under a psychological delusion.

At the same time, living with vulvodynia can be emotionally demanding, and it's completely understandable to feel anxious or depressed as a result of your vulvodynia. In fact, it's common. These feelings can even linger after the pain has been eliminated or greatly reduced [9]. In a later chapter, we'll discuss options and practices for coping with the emotional health side of vulvodynia.

Myth: Vulvodynia is linked to sexual abuse

Research has not uncovered any link between vulvodynia and sexual abuse. While it's true that vulvar pain may sometimes be triggered or aggravated by sexual intercourse, it is not caused by incidents of sexual abuse in the sufferer's past. Again, this is a dangerous myth that only stigmatizes women's health further. Of course, sexual abuse carries its own emotional scars. Visiting a licensed therapist can help victims of sexual abuse approach healing [9].

What is the Prognosis (Outlook) for Vulvodynia?

"With proper treatment, sufferers can lead normal, healthy lives that include good sex" [8].

Healing from vulvodynia may take several weeks or months, and treatment may not completely eliminate all symptoms. But through a combination of treatments and positive lifestyle changes, you can manage vulvodynia instead of letting it manage you [10]. The most important thing to keep in mind is that, "It doesn't have to last forever" [9].

Taking the First Step to Find Out What's Wrong

"An accurate diagnosis is half the battle, so now you can focus your efforts on finding helpful treatments and feeling better" [15]

Some women who experience vulvar pain discover that they are simply allergic to certain detergents, soaps, or other products. Or, they may have a vulvar skin condition or vaginal infection. If you think you may have an allergy, experiment with discontinuing the use of certain products to see if it helps. If you experience a vaginal infection which despite treatment, either disappears and then returns, or never goes away, you should make an appointment with your doctor [14].

Your doctor may want to screen you for sexually transmitted infections, depending on your risk factors and symptoms. They may also want to determine if you have vulvar itch or increased vaginal discharge, which could indicate a condition called vulvovaginal candidiasis. Since vulvar pain, which makes sexual intercourse painful and uncomfortable, can contribute to sexual dysfunction, your doctor may also consider sexual dysfunction as a related condition, though sexual dysfunction is not the cause of vulvodynia, but a possible result [16].

Because vulvodynia is such a misunderstood condition, you'll want to get a full assessment, including a thorough examination and analysis of your complete medical and sexual history, performed by a doctor or clinician who specializes in vulvar pain. A specialist should be able to diagnose your pain and rule out or identify any underlying causes. Doctors who specialize in vulvodynia can include gynecologists, GUM physicians, dermatologists, pain physicians, and urologists.

Your doctor should be open about the fact that no single vulvodynia treatment is effective. In other words, they should explain to you that you'll likely need to try a number of treatment methods, and may need to combine multiple treatments, to start managing your pain. They should adopt an individualized approach to your care, and guide you through the process of finding an effective solution. They may also point you to support groups, which as we'll discuss later, can be extremely helpful [3].

Chapter 2

Understanding the Basics

Diagnosing vulvodynia can take time. Every case is different, and there is a wide variety of symptoms, ranging from mild to incapacitating [1].

While it's hard to be patient when you're experiencing pain or frustrating symptoms, the truth is it will simply take time for your doctor to rule out all the possible causes of your vulvar pain and identify your specific type of vulvodynia. After that, it will take time for you and your doctor to pin down the right treatment and therapy options for your condition.

There are many different treatment and therapy options available for vulvodynia, and what works for some women may not work for you. Keep this in mind as you seek treatment and try not to get discouraged when something doesn't work. With the help of your doctor or clinician, you can simply move on to the next option, realizing that you're one step closer to relief.

Once you find a successful approach, don't despair if it takes longer than expected for relief to come. While you should definitely tell your doctor if you think a treatment is ineffective, progress can often be slow with vulvodynia. Instead of anxiously awaiting the day when you'll be completely pain-free, focus on getting a little better every day. Keeping a positive outlook can be challenging, but it's the best way forward.

The Basics of Vulvovaginal Anatomy

"Most women do not understand vulvovaginal anatomy and it certainly doesn't help that parts below the belly button are usually referred to as "down there" [1].

As the National Vulvodynia Association states, "It is important to participate in treatment decisions and discuss your progress with your doctor or health care provider. You know more about how you feel than anyone else" [1]. Having a basic understanding of vulvovaginal anatomy can help you communicate with your doctor.

Getting up Close and Personal

Your mouth and lips are interconnected, but are often referred to as two different things. And in health care, we don't treat the mouth and lips as one and the same. For example, "If you have chapped lips, you apply lip balm to the surface of your lips and not inside your mouth. The same applies to a vulvar disorder, i.e., you don't insert medicine into the vagina to treat a condition of the external tissue" [1]. Just as we distinguish between the mouth and lips, we also distinguish between the vulva and vagina, which are composed of different tissues. If you receive a diagnosis of a vaginal disorder, such as a bacterial or yeast infection, you need to place medicine into your vagina [1].

The Perineum

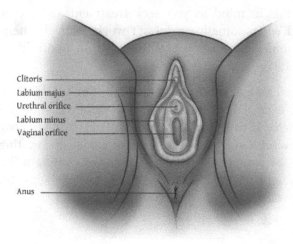

Clitoris

Labium majus

Urethral orifice

Labium minus

Vaginal orifice

Anus

The perineum, which is found between the pubic symphysis (a joint made of cartilage near the clitoris), and the coccyx (a small triangular bone at the bottom of the spine), is situated between the legs and below the pelvic diaphragm. In women, this is a diamond-shaped area which includes the vagina and anus. The perineum plays a crucial role in functions including sexual intercourse, micturition, defecation, and childbirth [1].

The Female Genitalia

The Vulva

The vulva refers to the external part of the female genitalia. Its functions include protecting the vestibule, urinary opening, and vagina. Directly above the vulva is the tissue covering the pubic bone, known as the mons pubis. The vulva's outer and inner 'lips' are known as the labia majora and labia minora, respectively. Situated above the opening to the vagina is the clitoris [1].

The vagina opening, and the opening of the urethra, are surrounded by the vestibule. The vagina and the vulva contain different tissue. The vagina passageway starts at the opening of the vagina and ends at the cervix, inside the body at the lowest part of the uterus. The bladder is situated straight in front of the vagina, and the rectum is found behind it. The vagina's length and width vary between women [1].

The Vagina

The vagina comprises tissue which can expand and contract. It has various functions, including stopping harmful bacteria from entering the body, facilitating sexual intercourse, and expanding during childbirth [1].

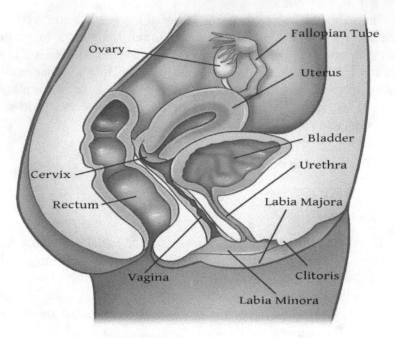

The Pudendal Nerve

The pudendal nerve starts at the sacral spine, which is found directly below the low back. It passes through the pelvis and then goes into the vulvar area, close to the ischial spine (which forms part of the pelvis). It then divides into the inferior rectal nerve, perineal nerve, and dorsal nerve of the clitoris. In both men and women, it is the pudendal nerve which is responsible for orgasm, correct functioning, and control of urination and defecation [1].

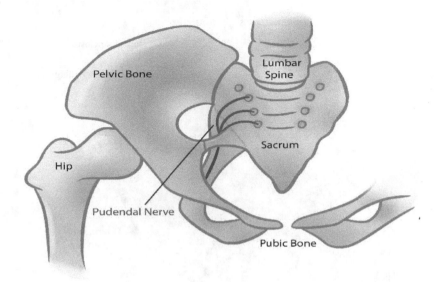

The Pelvic Floor Muscles

The pelvic floor comprises pelvic muscles, tendons, ligaments, and nerves. Strong pelvic floor muscles are essential for trunk mobility and stability, and function cooperatively to enable sexual, bowel, and bladder function. The pelvic floor muscles are separated into two types: the superficial muscles (collectively referred to as the urogenital triangle); and the deep muscles (the anal triangle). Other related muscles are the piriformis and the obturator internus [1].

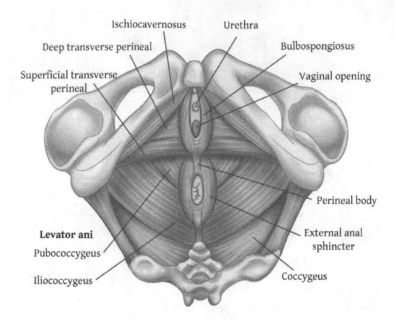

Vulvar Texture and Skin Color

The outer lips, or labia majora, defend the inner regions of the vulva, and the color of the outer lips is akin to your overall skin tone. The outer lips house a large number of oil-secreting and sweat glands and pubic hair. Below the lips, a layer of fat protects and cushions the region during sexual intercourse.

The inner lips, or labia minora, are located between the outer lips, and their color varies from deep pink to reddish, brownish pink. They may be thick, bumpy bulges, or thin, small flaps [1].

The inner lips' surface is moist and smooth, with glands situated along the edges. The glands look like tiny pimples, with a pebbly appearance. The tissue around the vaginal opening (the vestibule), is found at the base of the inner lips. This tissue is pink and moist, although on occasions, it can look almost red. The clitoris (which is cloaked by a retractable hood) sits above the urethra, where the inner lips converge [1].

Understanding Vulvovaginal Symptoms

Every woman's vulva looks different, and vaginal odor and secretions also differ. As the National Vulvodynia Association explains, "Sometimes it is difficult to figure out which characteristics are normal, and which are not. If you notice any abnormalities, consult your health care provider promptly and resist the temptation to self-treat" [1]. This advice of not self-treating cannot be overstated. As soon as you notice any concerning symptoms, book an appointment with your doctor.

Be Aware of Changes

From time to time, you may experience color changes or bumps in the vulva region. These may indicate a problem, or they may be completely harmless. In any case, if you notice color changes or bumps, make an appointment to see your doctor [1].

Vaginal Discharge

You may sometimes notice vaginal discharge, or fluid from your vagina that ranges from watery to a texture like milk or glue. Experiencing some vaginal discharge is completely normal. It's caused by a number of factors, such as specialized gland secretions (including Skene's and Bartholin's); mucus from the cervix; and cells cast off from the walls of the vagina. Vaginal discharge is mildly acidic, and helps protect the vagina from infection [1].

The amount of discharge fluctuates according to your hormonal status, increasing midway through the cycle at the time of ovulation and right afterwards. Throughout your menstrual cycle, the discharge color also changes, ranging from clear to slightly yellow or milky white [1].

If you're on oral contraceptives, you may have a different experience. Because the pill keeps your hormones' estrogen and progesterone levels steady, it also keeps your vaginal discharge from changing throughout the month.

In terms of your amount of discharge, what is normal for your body is different for everyone.

The National Vulvodynia Association advises, "It is important to remember that normal secretions do not itch, burn or irritate, nor do they smell like fish or ammonia. Abnormal discharge varies in its amount and appearance. Secretions may become more profuse, cause a strong odor, change in color (from clear to gray-white, yellow-white or yellow-green), and/or contain traces of blood, if inflammation is severe" [1]. If you notice any of these symptoms, contact your doctor.

Odor

"Each woman has a unique scent" [1].

The vulva contains many sweat-producing glands that give off odor and enable heat to escape. You don't need to worry if your vulvovaginal area emits an odor. But if the odor is unusually strong, you may want to talk to your doctor.

A strong, abnormal odor may be a sign of vaginal inflammation or vaginitis. BV (bacterial vaginosis) is thought to be the main culprit. It raises the vagina's usually acidic pH, thus generating a smell of dead fish (in severe cases), or in milder cases, ammonia. A fishy smell can also be brought on by Trichomoniasis (a sexually transmitted disease caused by a parasite). A less common reason for suffering an unpleasant odor is yeast infection. [1]. In any case, an unpleasant odor is no cause for alarm, and your doctor should be able to treat it.

Alternately, your vulvovaginal area may not have an odor at all. This simply means that your vaginal secretions are normal. Normal secretions may also have an odor that fluctuates throughout the course of the menstrual cycle or smells like sour milk [1].

Changes during Pregnancy and Childbirth

During pregnancy, your vaginal secretions may turn a violet-bluish color, increase, and/or have a thicker consistency. If you are pregnant and your discharge becomes watery, this could indicate that your cervix has weakened, generating leakage. If this happens, contact your doctor. Some women experience uncomfortable varicose veins within the vulvar region [1].

If your baby is delivered via the vagina, your vagina will temporarily expand. You may have a visible perineal scar (between the vaginal opening and the anus) if a tear or episiotomy occurs at the time of delivery, but this is nothing to worry about.

Estrogen levels are extremely low during the postpartum period. This is especially true for women who breastfeed their babies, and low estrogen can substantially reduce vaginal lubrication, or the naturally produced fluid that keeps your vagina smooth and free of friction. To help protect the vulva after giving birth, it's a good idea to refrain from sexual intercourse for a minimum of four to six weeks [1].

Changes during Menopause

During the five to ten years prior to menopause (known as the perimenopausal period), you may experience an increase in bacterial or yeast infections, vaginal itchiness or dryness, and/or discomfort during intercourse. Because of the reduction in estrogen during the perimenopausal period, the skin of the vulva becomes drier and thinner, making intercourse uncomfortable. The opening of the vagina can seem smaller due to the inner lips shrinking or flattening. In addition, vaginal discharge can vanish or become minimal unless women take certain medications such as tamoxifen, are overweight, or on hormone replacement therapy [1].

If you experience any menopause-related discomfort, contact your doctor for advice. There's a myth that pain and discomfort during menopause is just something women have to tolerate, but the truth is, there are plenty of treatments and therapies that can minimize uncomfortable menopause symptoms.

Vulva Self-Examination (VSE)

"All sexually active women, and women over 18 years old, should perform a vaginal self-examination" [1].

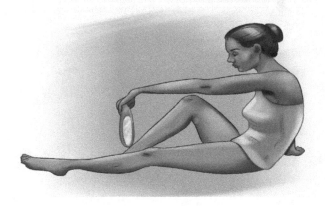

Many women perform breast self-examinations, but only a small percentage have heard about the importance of VSE (vulva self-examination). The National Vulvodynia Association advises that "you should perform VSE to detect abnormalities that may indicate infection or disease" [1] between routine gynecological examinations. "It is important to start performing VSE at an early age, so you can learn what is normal and then recognize any changes. You should not experience discomfort from your VSE, unless you have an infection, open sore or other vulvar condition" [1].

How Do I Perform a VSE?

Choose a room that has good lighting, preferably daylight. Wash your hands before and after. You can either stand with one foot on a bed or sturdy chair, or sit where you have room to maneuver. Hold a mirror in one hand so you can see into your vulva, keeping the other hand free to make the examination [1].

Look at and touch all the regions of your vulva. These include the skin around the opening of the vagina, the left and right folds of the outer and inner lips, the clitoris and its surrounding area, the mons pubis, the perineum, and the perianal region [1].

What Am I looking For?

The National Vulvodynia Association suggests things to look for during your VSE:

- "Do you see a new mole, wart, lump or other growth?

- Is there a change in skin color, e.g., white, reddened, or brown patches?

- Are there any cuts or sores?

- Is there a change in the way the vulvar skin feels?" [1].

Apply gentle pressure all around the skin to check for any lumps. Pay close attention to any areas of concern, such as those that are giving you discomfort, itching, stinging, or pain [1].

How Often Should I Conduct a VSE?

Conduct this self-examination once a month. If you have periods, it's best to do a VSE midway through your cycle. If you notice anything you think maybe abnormal during your VSE, contact your doctor [1].

Chapter 3

Getting a Diagnosis

According to the National Institutes of Health (NIH) "Vulvodynia tends to be diagnosed only when other causes of vulvar pain, such as infection or skin diseases, have been ruled out" [1].

"Each woman needs an individualized assessment and intervention plan that addresses the specific biological, psychological, and social factors contributing to her pain, and the impact of her pain on her life" [2]

Before your doctor diagnoses you with vulvodynia, they will go through your medical, surgical, and sexual history in detail so they can understand your situation. They will also ask you various questions about the nature, whereabouts, and intensity of your symptoms, including pain characteristics and any sexual, bowel, or bladder issues that you are experiencing. The more in-depth, descriptive information you can give, the better [1,3].

Following is some of the information your doctor will ask about. By knowing what to expect, you can go in prepared and help speed up the diagnosis process.

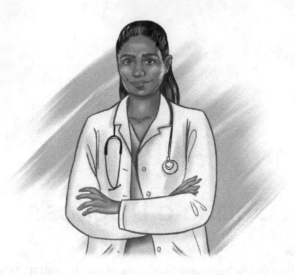

20 Questions

Your doctor will likely ask you many questions about your pain, your symptoms, your sexual life, and more. While this part can be tedious, try to be patient and answer the questions as accurately as possible. Your doctor needs all the information you can provide in order to give you an accurate diagnosis.

Pain Level, Triggers, and Descriptors

Your doctor will ask you several questions about the onset of your condition. For example: is the pain spontaneous or provoked? Do certain activities aggravate it? They may try to find out if your pain has been caused by a trigger, such as candidiasis or another infection, having a gynecological examination, long periods of sitting down, riding a bicycle, inserting a tampon, or intercourse [4]. If you experience frequent vulvar pain, it may be useful to keep a daily record to show your doctor.

You will also be asked to describe your pain in as much detail as possible. (This is another useful thing to record daily.) Your doctor may ask if your pain feels like a stinging, sharp, or burning sensation. They may also ask if you suffer from pruritis (an unpleasant itching sensation of the skin). Other questions include what improves the pain, your degree of pain, and the effect of the pain on your quality of life [4]. Finally, you will be asked whether the pain is localized (confined to a single area) or generalized (all over).

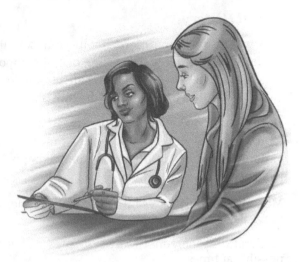

Overlapping Symptoms

Your doctor may want to know if you have noticed any skin lesions (color changes, ulcers, or skin masses on the vulva), which could indicate vulvar intraepithelial neoplasia or vulvar dermatoses.

They will also check for signs of overlapping conditions. For example: fibromyalgia (general body pain); irritable bowel syndrome (bloating, diarrhea, constipation, abdominal pain); low back pain; or painful bladder syndrome (urgency, bladder pain, pelvic pain) [4]. Any of these conditions could cause or be related to your vulvar pain.

Other relevant conditions include genital nerve injury, spine or hip surgery, vulvovaginal or pelvic surgeries, herpes zoster and herpes simplex. Your doctor may also ask if you are experiencing co-morbid (coexisting) conditions like stress, depression, anxiety, interstitial cystitis, chronic low back pain, fibromyalgia, or irritable bowel syndrome.

Treatment History

If you've received treatment for vulvodynia or related conditions in the past, your doctor will want to know about it. You should tell them when you began each therapy or treatment, how long you continued with it, what dosage of medications you were prescribed, whether or not you took the medication, any side-effects you experienced, and the reason your treatment stopped (if relevant) [4].

Psychosexual History

Your doctor will also ask questions about your sexual history. While you may feel uncomfortable discussing this, it's important for your doctor to know whether your vulvodynia affects and/or is tied to your sexual life so they can give an accurate diagnosis.

Your doctor will ask how often you have sex, what percentage of the time you enjoy it, and what percentage of the time you experience pain or discomfort with sex. Painful sexual intercourse is known as dyspareunia, and occurs on three levels:

- Mild dyspareunia- present most of the time, does not prevent sexual intercourse

- Moderate dyspareunia- always present, intercourse possible at times

- Severe dyspareunia- prohibits intercourse [4]

In addition to asking about your current and past sexual experiences, your doctor will want to know whether you have a history of vaginismus (spasmodic contraction of the vagina in response to pressure or physical contact, particularly during sexual relations) [4].

Finally, you may be asked if you have any history of physical, emotional, or sexual abuse. Again, this is not a fun topic to discuss, but it's important information for your doctor to have so they can diagnose and treat you correctly.

Physical Assessment

"Pelvic examination and localization of the symptoms and signs to the area of the vestibule differentiates localized vulvodynia (LVD) from other causes of vulvar pain" [4].

Pelvic Exam

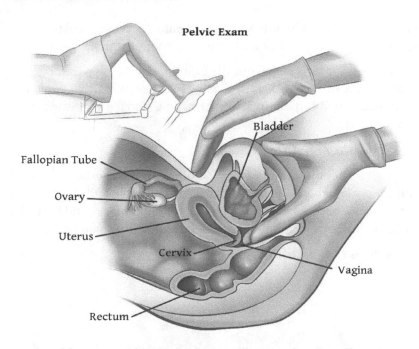

Fallopian Tube

Ovary

Uterus

Cervix

Rectum

Bladder

Vagina

In addition to asking you questions, your doctor will perform a physical examination. This involves a pelvic exam, in which your doctor will examine your vagina and vulva to see if you have an infection or skin disorder (such as lichen sclerosis and lichen planus) [4], or whether your symptoms are due to other causes [1,3].

The doctor will look for any signs of sores, cuts, skin picking, red skin, or abnormally light skin in the vulva region, so that vulvar skin defects and vulvovaginal infection can be ruled out [4]. Even if a visual infection is not evident, your doctor may still test for bacterial vaginosis, a yeast infection, or other common disorders by taking a simple, painless cell sample [1,3]. They may also suggest blood work to determine your levels of estrogen, progesterone, and testosterone [1]. Other tests may be carried out to rule out peripheral neuropathy (dysfunctional nerves in the body's extremities), and test for menopause or perimenopause (being around the time of menopause).

While these physical examinations should not be painful under normal circumstances, they can be for women suffering from vulvodynia. In some assessments, your doctor may test specifically for pain, but even then, an experienced provider will be sensitive to your discomfort and do what they can to minimize your discomfort. They may use a local anesthetic to reduce discomfort or use a small pediatric speculum to visually check for erosions, atrophy, or fibrous scars [4].

If you are concerned about the examination being painful, share that concern with your doctor. Finally, just remember that while the examination may be painful, it won't last long, and it's a necessary step toward relief.

Screening for Infections

To screen for infections, your doctor may use bacterial and fungal cultures, vaginal pH, and wet smears. This helps them rule out vulvovaginal infections like candidiasis, trichomoniasis, and bacterial vaginosis—all of which can be associated with vulvar pain [4].

A Moistened Cotton Swab Test

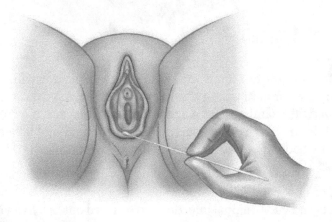

Some doctors will use a moistened cotton swab to gently check your vulva for localized areas where you experience pain. As your doctor applies gentle pressure to various parts of your vulva, they will ask you to rate your level of pain, for example, on a scale of 1 to 10. If any regions seem abnormally painful, your doctor may use a magnifying instrument to take a closer look, or, in rare cases, they may take a tissue biopsy or other test [1,3].

Digital Examination

In a digital examination, the doctor uses one finger to gauge the pelvic floor muscle tone, check for tenderness, and evaluate how well your pelvic floor muscles function. They also check for any masses:

lumps caused by a cyst, hormonal change, immune reaction, or abnormal cell growth.

Vulvar Biopsy

In most cases, your doctor will not need to perform a vulvar biopsy. This may only be necessary if your symptoms suggest intraepithelial neoplasia (the development of abnormal cells in the surface layers of the skin covering the vulva), or vulvar dermatoses, or if your case is unclear and additional pathology is suspected [4].

Can an MRI scan Help?

An MRI (magnetic resonance imaging) scan of the pelvis may help to rule out any obvious pelvic abnormalities. If your doctor thinks an MRI would be helpful, they may choose to examine the following:

- Pelvic viscera (organs)
- Bilateral pudendal nerves
- Bilateral sacral nerve roots
- Bone and soft tissues of the pelvis and hips

Do Vulvodynia Sufferers Often Have the Same Additional Health Problems?

Conditions like fibromyalgia, painful bladder syndrome (also known as interstitial cystitis), irritable bowel syndrome, low back pain, anxiety, and depression are frequent among vulvodynia sufferers [5].

Choose Your Doctor with Care

"**Women typically consult with three or more physicians before obtaining an accurate diagnosis. Even once a diagnosis is reached, ongoing involvement with medical professionals commonly persists because of the limited benefit of medicinal treatments**" **[4].**

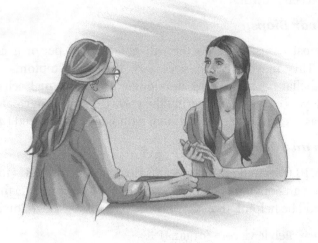

Not every doctor or clinician is experienced in diagnosing and treating vulvodynia. When choosing a doctor, take your time to thoroughly research the available options. Look at reviews, ratings, and credentials to find a doctor who has an excellent track record.

Be mindful of the fact that all knowledgeable vulvovaginal specialists and gynecologists undertake a careful examination, test for all skin diseases, fungal and bacterial infections [6], and give a clear explanation of their diagnosis, as well as useful information for you to take home [4]. If you feel that your doctor is not qualified or is not doing a good job, you may want to seek a second opinion.

Toward Treatment

"Multimodal therapy should be part of the treatment strategy because the cause of the condition can be due to multiple factors" [4].

Whatever your type of vulvodynia, your doctor's initial goal is to decrease vulvar irritation and pain through appropriate care. Most patients benefit from a combination of counseling, pelvic floor physical therapy, topical or oral medications, and occasionally surgery.

The goal of any treatment methods will be to "optimize pain control, enhance psychological and physical well-being, and improve quality of life. The end points in the treatment include reducing the triggers of irritation, blocking peripheral pain receptors, central inhibition, tackling pelvic floor dysfunction and addressing psychosexual dysfunction" [4].

If your doctor recommends a multidisciplinary approach [7,8], you may need an appointment with a pelvic floor physical therapist (or physiotherapist), a psychosexual medicine specialist (psychiatrist, psychologist, or sex therapist), and a referral to a pain management specialist.

Chapter 4

Vulva Self-Help Tips

Caring for your vulva is essential to good health and can sometimes help to lessen vulvar pain. To review, the vulva lies outside the vagina, and is comprised of the following: the labia (folds of tissue, which are sometimes referred to as the "lips"), namely the labia majora (the outermost folds); and the labia minora (the innermost folds on each side of the opening of the vagina); the mons pubis (the mounded area over the pubic bone); the clitoris (a small, round organ); and the opening of the vagina and urethra.

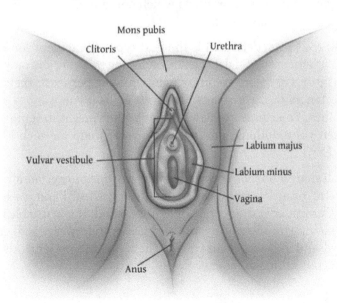

The Goal

In caring for your vulva, the prime goal is to keep it dry and free from irritants. Doing so will promote healthy vulva skin and prevent the area from becoming irritated, swollen, and red. As several infections can enter the body directly through the vagina, keeping the vulvar area clean and dry goes a long way toward optimum health for your vulva, vagina, and whole body. Following the tips in this chapter will help you maintain good vulvar and vaginal health [1,2].

Guidelines for Good Vulvar Health

To care for your vulva, you'll want to remove or decrease moisture, chemicals, and friction. The following tips can help relieve or decrease vulvar/vaginal itching, irritation, and burning [2], keeping your vulva healthy and safe.

Laundry

The laundry products and washing machine settings you use can affect your vulvar health. Detergents that claim to improve, brighten, or whiten your laundry usually use harsh chemicals that can cause itchiness and irritation. Bleach, dryer sheets, and fabric softeners can dry out your skin, as can products which contain enzymes (cellulose, protease, lipase, or amylase).

"All Free Clear" detergent is the best type of detergent for vulvar health. With most special detergents, including this one, you only need to use 1/3 or 1/2 of the recommended amount per load. Instead of fabric softeners or dryer sheets, use dryer balls if you want to soften your clothes. You can use lemon juice or white vinegar to remove oils or freshen your clothing, putting in 1/4 to 1/3 cup for each load of laundry [2,3].

If you share a washer or dryer, such as in a dormitory, laundromat, launderette, or apartment, always use All Free Clear hand wash, and air dry your underwear on a line or clothes stand. If you use bleach or stain-removing products on any towels or underwear, soak them afterward and rinse in clean water. Then wash them with All Free Clear on your normal washing cycle.

In summary

Avoid the following:

- Detergents that use harsh chemicals to improve, brighten, or whiten your laundry

- Bleach

- Dryer sheets

- Fabric softeners

- Products that contain enzymes

Use these instead:

- All Free Clear detergent

- 1/2 to 1/3 of recommended detergent amount per load

- Dryer balls

- Lemon juice or white vinegar (1/3 to 1/4 cup per load)

- Air dry underwear instead of using a shared dryer

- After bleaching laundry, soak, rinse, and wash it

Clothing

Underwear is constantly in contact with your vulva, and as such, you need to make sure you're only choosing the best, healthiest types of underclothes. Only use all-white, 100% cotton underwear that has a good-sized cotton (not nylon) crotch. Always wash new underclothes before wearing them.

Nylon, acetate, and other man-made fiber underwear is not breathable. Only cotton lets the skin breathe by allowing air to circulate. It also keeps moisture away from the vulva. Heat and moisture provide an ideal environment for infectious organisms.

When you go to bed, never wear thongs or underwear. Cotton pajama bottoms work fine, as do loose-fitting female cotton boxers.

Tight clothing is not your vulva's friend. Avoid clothing that's too tight around your crotch, especially tight clothing that contains synthetic fabrics. Opt for stockings or thigh-high hose rather than tights. If you do wear tights, and they do not have a cotton gusset, you can cut the diamond crotch away, and in order to prevent running, leave around 1/4 inch of material from the seam.

After exercising or swimming, always take off exercise gear and damp or wet bathing clothes as soon as possible [2,3].

In summary

Avoid the following:

- Nylon, acetate, or man-made fiber underwear
- Tight underwear
- Tights
- Wearing underwear or thongs at night

Use these instead:

- All-white, 100% cotton underwear
- Stockings or thigh-high tights
- Cotton pajama bottoms or loose-fitting cotton boxers

Hygiene and Bathing

When it comes to hygiene and bathing, you can't be too careful about how you treat your vulva and what you allow to come into contact with it. First of all, take any baths or showers at a moderate temperature. If the water is too cold or too hot, it can irritate your skin.

The best soaps include Pears, Aveeno, Basis, Neutrogena, and Dove for Sensitive Skin. Even when using one of these soaps, however, never use soap directly on the skin of the vulva. Avoid using a loofah, body brush, washcloth, sponge, or anything else to scrub the vulva skin. Simply washing your vulvar region with warm water by hand prevents irritation and is sufficient to keep the vulva clean. The vagina naturally cleanses itself through normal vaginal discharge, so you don't need to worry too much about cleaning it manually.

Never use a douche. To dispel odor and any discharge, simply rinse the region using warm water or baking soda soaks.

Never use any form of hair removal products or shave the vulva region. Laser treatment may be an option (subject to any contra-indications); and any pubic hair growing in the vulva region can simply be trimmed with scissors, provided the scissors have been cleaned with surgical spirit (for example, rubbing alcohol) prior to use.

Washing your hair while in the shower can cause the shampoo to flow down to the vulvar region. Because of this, it's important to always rinse the vulva extremely well after washing your hair so there are no traces of shampoo left.

Avoid using any type of perfumed feminine hygiene products, feminine sprays, gels, lotions, creams, bath soaps, scrubs, and so on. Similarly, never use scented oils, bath salts, or bubble bath. Always read the product labels before you make a purchase, as even bath and shower items which are touted as mild, gentle, natural, and organic may contain added perfume. While they may smell lovely, these products can cause irritation, which can lead to further issues.

Avoid putting body lotion directly on the vulva. When you exit the shower or bathtub, and your skin is still damp, you can apply a neutral (unperfumed, unscented) lotion or oil to the area around the vulva. But remember that the skin must be damp, and remember not to directly apply the lotion to the vulva.

Only use white, 100% cotton towels and washcloths, and be sure to keep your washcloth and towel separate from those belonging to other people in your household. Never use a towel, cloth, or similar item to rub the vulva dry. Instead, either blow cool air from a hair dryer or just pat the region dry with a very soft towel or cloth.

In summary

Avoid the following:

- Scalding hot or freezing cold water
- Soap or lotion directly on the skin of the vulva
- A douche
- Scrubbing the vulva skin
- Hair removal products for the vulva region
- Shaving the vulva
- Perfumed feminine hygiene products
- Scented oils, bath salts, or bubble bath

- Body lotion directly on the vulva
- Rubbing the vulva with a towel or cloth

Use these instead:

- Lukewarm water
- Pears, Aveeno, Basis, Neutrogena, and Dove for Sensitive Skin soap
- Warm water or baking soda soaks to clean the vulva
- Sanitized scissors to trim vulvar hair
- Neutral lotion or oil to the area around the vulva
- White, 100% cotton towels and washcloths
- To dry: blow cool air from a hair dryer or pat dry

Toilet Paper, Pads, and Tampons

Toilet paper, pads, tampons, and other feminine hygiene products serve to protect the vulva and vagina from infection. But using the wrong products, or even using the right products in the wrong way, can be detrimental.

Only use soft white, unscented toilet paper. Don't use aloe-softened toilet paper. Many toilet paper brands contain perfume, so be aware of this, and be sure to check the package ingredients before purchase. Do not buy recycled toilet paper, as the recycling process uses harsh chemicals.

When you go to the toilet, always wipe yourself from the front to the back, and pat your vulva region dry instead of wiping. Avoid using baby wipes or adult wipes.

Only choose pads that have a liner made of pure cotton, as this part of the pad contacts the vulva. Never use ones with a nylon mesh or dry weave plastic lining, as these retain moisture, keeping discharge and blood next to your skin longer. Recommended brands include Stayfree, Seventh Generation, or Kotex.

Never wear deodorized pads or tampons, except on occasion when you experience heavy blood flow that could soak a tampon within four hours. In this case, it's OK to insert a deodorized tampon for limited use.

For most women, tampons are safe, as long as they're not kept inserted for too long. Leaving them in for too long can bring on odor, increased discharge, vaginal infection, or toxic shock syndrome. Always change your tampons, pads, and sanitary towels frequently, and never leave any kind of tampon in overnight.

If you suffer from incontinence, only purchase protective pads specifically made for incontinence and designed to absorb urine. You will most likely experience less skin irritation, and have less odor, than you would if you used sanitary pads for menstrual blood. Only put the protective pads onto clean skin.

If you need to use hemorrhoid pads, then the Trucks brand is recommended.

In summary

Avoid the following:

- Scented or aloe-softened toilet paper
- Recycled toilet paper
- Baby wipes or adult wipes
- Pads with a nylon mesh or dry weave plastic lining
- Deodorized pads or tampons
- Leaving a tampon in overnight

Use/Do these instead:

- Soft white unscented toilet paper
- Wipe from front to back, patting vulva region dry
- Pads with a pure cotton liner
- Stayfree, Seventh Generation, or Kotex pads
- Trucks hemorrhoid pads

Protecting the Vulva

When it comes to protecting your vulva from moisture and irritation, there are plenty of steps you can take at home.

Always consult your health care provider before you put on any over-the-counter ointments or creams. Only buy fragrance-free ointments that do not contain parabens. Have a good look at the label, as they are often very long, and these components can be hard to spot.

If you need to protect your vulva skin, just dab on a small amount of plain unscented Vaseline, zinc oxide ointment, vegetable oil, coconut oil, or extra virgin olive oil as frequently as necessary to ensure that the skin is protected. Only purchase good quality oil, preferably in a glass bottle. This process will help to reduce any skin irritation that you may experience when you urinate, or during the time of your period.

If you feel a burning sensation in your skin from urine, then as you urinate, pour lukewarm water from a plastic jug over the vulva region. Remember not to wipe the area dry; only pat.

Baking soda soaks can help reduce vulvar burning and itching. Fill your bath with lukewarm water and add 4 to 5 tablespoons of baking soda. Before stepping in, ensure that the bath water is lukewarm. This treatment can be carried out between once and three times per day.

You can also use a sitz bath to get the same results. A sitz bath or hip bath is a bath in which a person sits in water up to the hips. It's used to relieve discomfort and pain in the lower part of the body. Just add 1 to 2 teaspoons of baking soda to lukewarm bath water.

If you are experiencing an irritation or itch in the vulva region, avoid swimming pools, Jacuzzis, and hot tubs. All three use harsh chemicals to kill bacteria [2,3].

Keeping your vulva dry is essential, especially if you suffer from long-term dampness. To keep your vulva dry, always carry spare underwear with you; that way, you can change whenever you become damp. Always purchase 100% cotton fabrics as opposed to other materials, including those mixed with cotton. Avoid wearing pads every day when not menstruating. In order to help your skin absorb moisture, apply Zeasorb powder or Gold Bond all around the groin and vulva region once or twice per day. Just be sure not to use any powder that contains cornstarch.

Never scratch your genital area. Avoid crossing your legs and do not stay sitting down for a long time. Never use a waterbed, electric blanket, or plastic mattress cover.

In summary

Avoid the following:

- Products that contain parabens
- Wearing pads every day when not menstruating
- Powder that contains cornstarch
- Scratching your genital area
- Crossing your legs
- Sitting for long periods of time
- Waterbeds, electric blankets, or plastic mattress covers

Use these instead:

- Plain unscented Vaseline, zinc oxide ointment, vegetable oil, coconut oil, or extra virgin olive oil
- Lukewarm water, baking soda soaks, and sitz baths
- Zeasorb powder or Gold Bond
- Spare underwear to keep the vulva dry

Sexual Intercourse

In order to protect your vulva during and after sex, follow these tips for hygiene and lubrication.

To help flush away any germs that may have entered your bladder or urethra, empty your bladder after sexual intercourse. This will help prevent bladder infections. Always wash and dry the vulva region after you have had sexual intercourse. If you use a "sex toy," vaginal dilator, or diaphragm, clean it thoroughly with mild soap and water after use. Then rinse and dry completely.

Moustaches, beards, and saliva can cause irritation. If you have had any form of anal contact, avoid genital contact afterwards.

You can reduce irritation and dryness during intercourse by using a lubricant. Dispense a small amount of natural pure vegetable oil (liquid, solid, extra virgin olive oil, or coconut), and use your middle finger to insert it into your vagina. As these products do not contain any added chemicals, they shouldn't irritate your vaginal/vulvar skin. Plus, your chances of infection will not increase if you use vegetable oils, and they can be easily rinsed away with water.

It might also help to use a non-spermicidal, non-lubricated condom (which is not needed for birth control or protection against sexual diseases) along with the vegetable oil lubricant. This may lessen any irritation and burning after intercourse, as it can help to stop semen contacting the skin [2].

Avoid the water-based lubricants available over the counter, as they may use chemicals that can irritate the genital skin. These lubricants tend to dry out during intercourse and may cause small tears in the vagina.

In summary

Avoid the following:

- Engaging in genital contact directly after anal contact
- Using a water-based, over-the-counter lubricant

Do these instead:

- Empty your bladder after sexual intercourse
- Wash and dry the vulva region after intercourse
- Wash, rinse, and dry sex toys after use
- Use a small amount of pure vegetable oil to lubricate

Birth Control

If you're using pills, contraceptive jellies, or condoms as a birth control method, it's important to separate fact from fiction so you can protect your vulva and your overall health.

As previously mentioned, you may be able to protect your skin by applying a vegetable/coconut oil lubricant and using latex condoms, unless you are latex-allergic. A lubricant that is both oil-based and petroleum-based, however, could affect the condom's integrity. So if you're using a condom to prevent sexually transmitted infections or pregnancy, using a vegetable/coconut oil lubricant is not recommended.

Sponges, creams, contraceptive jellies, and lubricated condoms have been known to cause burning and itching. If you have an allergy or sensitivity to contraceptive products, such as condoms, sponges, foams, mousses, or spermicides, see what other brands are available, and if necessary, consider changing your birth control method.

Your chance of contracting a yeast infection will not go up if you take low-dose oral birth control pills. Lastly, always notify your doctor about any new products you use on your vulva [2,3].

Chapter 5

Five Things Anyone with a Vagina Needs to Know

Recently, the BBC Health News channel published an article on the numerous false and misleading myths about the vagina (many circulating on social media), and the fact that help is hand. That BBC article, written by Dr. Jen Gunter [1], will help inform this chapter.

A One-Woman Mission

Dr. Gunter, a well-known North American obstetrician-gynecologist and a fierce exponent for women's health, is on a mission to give everyone with a vagina the right information. And she's doing extremely well. After 25 years in the field of women's intimate health, she has garnered the much-coveted title of Twitter's resident gynecologist. In her book, *The Vagina Bible*, Gunter works to empower women by giving them practical advice and health tips [1]. Let's look at some of her main points.

Number 1. Knowing Your Vagina from Your Vulva

At this point, let's review some basic anatomy. The vagina is inside the body; it's the inner muscular canal which links the uterus to the outside world. Conversely, the vulva touches women's clothes and can be seen from the outside. The vulva incorporates the outer parts around the vagina, including the vaginal lips, the clitoral hood, and the clitoris [1,2].

Rather than relying on euphemisms, Gunter notes that being au fait with the proper terminology is essential. "When you can't say the word vagina or vulva, there is an implication that there's something dirty or shameful about that." She points out that the medical term pudendal, which describes the outside of the vulva, comes from the Latin "pudet," meaning "it shames" [1].

Dr. Gunter believes that on an emotional level, if such labels are used, they can have negative mental connotations and even cause a poor medical outcome—simply because women do not have the correct vocabulary to describe their symptoms. In some cases, this can mean not being given the right treatment, or having to wait a long period of time until receiving the correct diagnosis [1].

Number 2. The Self-Cleansing Vagina

"Do you really need to wash your vagina? No, but you do need to wash your vulva" [2].

Have you ever used an intimate product to "beautify" the smell of your vagina? If you have, you're not alone. Gunter remarks that over the past decade she has witnessed an overwhelming trend in this direction. Many women share a collective belief that they need to use products to modify their vagina's smell. In fact, in the 12 months leading up to the publication of the BBC article, "up to 57% of women [in North America], have cleaned vaginally, with many reporting that they are encouraged to do so by their sexual partner" [1].

However, referring to the vagina as "a self-cleaning oven," Gunter insists that it is not necessary to use any products to clean inside the vagina [1]. "The American College of Obstetricians and Gynecologists points out that your vagina cleans itself and keeps itself healthy by maintaining the correct pH balance and cleaning itself with natural secretions" [2]. In other words, there's no need to clean your vagina.

"Your vagina contains a lot of 'good' bacteria" [1]

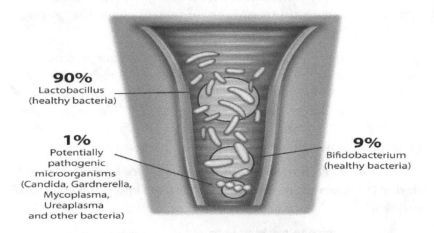

90%
Lactobacillus
(healthy bacteria)

1%
Potentially
pathogenic
microorganisms
(Candida, Gardnerella,
Mycoplasma,
Ureaplasma
and other bacteria)

9%
Bifidobacterium
(healthy bacteria)

The healthy bacteria in your vagina preserve its perfect pH balance, which is mildly acidic. This makes it difficult for the 'bad' bacteria to generate any infections in the region. But gels, sprays, soaps, and even water can disrupt this balance, potentially leading to irritations like yeast infections and bacterial vaginosis. Supermarkets and drug stores are awash (excuse the pun), with all kinds of perfumed intimate washes, and brand marketing seems to "prey on people's insecurities regarding their bodily odors" [2]. But it's not necessary to clean your vagina and/or eliminate its odor. Just say no!

Washing your vagina can also affect your vagina's ability to clean itself. So, if you want a clean vagina, leave it alone to clean itself! [2]

The perils of having a nice-smelling vagina are simply not worth it. For Gunter, scented douches are certainly on the "do not go there" list. She says, "it's a vagina, not a pina colada, douches are like cigarettes for your vagina" [1]. On another note, she points out that cleaning with water can upset the body's delicate ecosystem, which can raise the risk of acquiring sexually transmitted infections.

Another popular trend is steaming your vagina: something brought to the fore by Hollywood celebrities. Not only is this uncalled for, it can potentially burn a woman's delicate intimate tissues [1].

"Most supermarkets have a range of feminine washes & sprays that are said to reduce odor and clean the vagina. Don't buy these" [2].

When required, however, you can use water or a gentle pH balanced cleanser to clean the outside of the vulva region. Standard soap is not recommended, as it often removes the skin's protective waterproofing, known as the acid mantle. If the vagina feels uncomfortable and dry due to hormonal changes brought on by menopause, you might try applying olive oil or coconut oil [1].

"Vaginal cells are replaced every 96 hours—a much faster turnover than other parts of the skin—so it can heal quickly" [1].

When it comes to washing your vulva, you can use warm water, and if desired, a high quality, colorless, unscented, mild pH soap that won't irritate this sensitive region, although soap is not necessary. The most important thing is to use the right technique. Spread your vagina's lips apart, then, using your hands or a very soft, plain, unbleached white washcloth, gently clean around the folds [2].

Try not to get any soap or water inside your vagina. And remember to clean the anus, and the region between your vulva and anus, daily. Be sure to cleanse from the front to the back. In other words, start by washing the vulva, and then do the anus. If you wipe from back to front, bacteria from your anus can spread to your vagina, and you may end up with an infection [2].

Number 3. A Woman's Vagina is Like a Garden

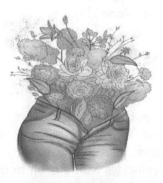

Gunter remarks that "The vaginal microbiome is like a garden of all different kinds of bacteria that function together to keep the vaginal ecosystem healthy" [1]. Apart from generating a mildly acidic surrounding, which prevents the bad bacteria taking hold, the vagina also produces mucus, which is essential for lubricating the region and for having sex. The myth that you should use omnipresent antibacterial wipes to clean the vagina is just that: a myth. These wipes can actually do more harm than good.

Number 4. Pubic Hair Does Have a Role

Gunter wants women to realize that pubic hair serves an important purpose. She condemns the popular "Full Brazilian" trend; or the process of waxing, shaving, sugaring, and lasering to remove all pubic hair. This process can cause more damage than just removing pubic hair, as these procedures can cause infections, abrasions, and cuts, as well as microscopic trauma to the skin. In particular, waxing operatives should not double-dip the wooden spatulas into the wax pot, as this can potentially spread harmful bacteria between customers [1]. Only certified practitioners should carry out such treatments.

In any case, women should carefully consider whether they want to take the Brazilian route. Gunter reiterates that "pubic hair has a function, that it is probably a mechanical barrier and protection for the skin, [and that] it may also have a role in sexual functioning, because each pubic hair is attached to a nerve ending—that's why it hurts to remove it" [1]. In light of this, shaving is not recommended.

But if women do want to shave, it's important to do it right. Always prepare the skin appropriately, use a clean single-blade razor, and shave in the direction of the growth of the hair to avoid ingrown hairs, which can easily become infected [1].

Number 5. The Vagina is Also Affected by Age

Just like most things, the vagina is subject to the wear and tear of age. After countless years of monthly periods, and for many women, years of having children, menstruation ends as the ovaries stop producing eggs. This coincides with a drop in the level of hormones that keep women fertile. Low levels of estrogen, especially, have a knock-on effect on the tissues of the vulva and vagina [1].

In fact, many women experience a cyclical variation in their vulvar pain due to hormones. If your oestrogen (one of the main female sex hormones) is low, you may find low dose testosterone helpful for relieving vulvodynia. Topical and oral oestrogens can help with this.

"You don't have to suffer" [1].

Before these changes, the tissues are constantly moistened by mucus; but age often leads to shriveling (atrophy) of the tissues, and it's normal to experience overriding dryness and lack of lubrication, resulting in painful sex. Certain over-the-counter lubricants (which if you have vulvodynia, should be recommended by your doctor) can improve the situation, and as long as you don't have any contra-indications, natural supplements may also help [1].

On a closing note, Gunter sums up a myth gleaned from poor research "there is a myth that having sex will help to keep things in working order, but the micro trauma to the vaginal tissues can leave them vulnerable to infection" [1].

Now that you're more familiar with your vulva and vagina, the role they play in your overall health, and the proper way to care for them, we'll move on in the next chapter to some common vulvodynia treatments.

Chapter 6

Summary of Treatment Options

There are many treatment options for vulvodynia, from simple steps like using different laundry or hygiene products, to more involved solutions like physical therapy or surgery. Recently, a group of doctors reviewed the medical research on vulvodynia from 1998 to 2013 in search of the best treatment options [1].

But as they discovered, the fact remains that there's no one-size-fits-all solution for treating vulvodynia. In light of this, the authors of the study suggest a multidisciplinary approach, combining topical and/or oral medications, dietary recommendations, biofeedback and physical therapy, self-care, and therapy and counseling. If this first approach fails to bring relief, the authors suggest a more involved plan that includes steps like steroid injections and pulsed radiofrequency treatment. If this second approach fails to bring relief, surgery may be required [1].

The different steps for treating vulvodynia according to this multidisciplinary approach are listed in the following chart "Proposed therapeutic algorithm model including an intermediate, minimally invasive stage for the treatment of vulvodynia [1]". We'll discuss many of them in more detail later.

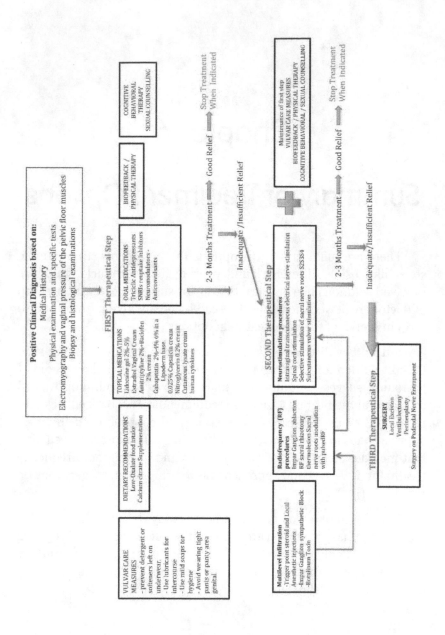

Positive Clinical Diagnosis based on:
Medical History
Physical examination and specific tests
Electromyography and vaginal pressure of the pelvic floor muscles
Biopsy and histological examinations

FIRST Therapeutical Step

VULVAR CARE MEASURES
- prevent detergent or softeners left on underwear.
- Use lubricants for intercourse
- Use mild soaps for hygiene
- Avoid wearing tight pants or panty area genital

DIETARY RECOMMENDATIONS
Low-Oxalate food intake
Calcium citrate Supplementation

TOPICAL MEDICATIONS
Lidocaine gel 2%-5%
Estradiol Vaginal Cream
Amitriptyline 2%+Baclofen 2% cream
Gabapentin 2%-4%-6% in a Lipoderm base.
0.025% Capsaicin cream
Nitroglycerin 0.2% cream
Cutaneous lysate cream human cytokines

ORAL MEDICATIONS
Triclcic Antidepressants
SNRIs reuptake inhibitors
Neuromodulators -
Anticonvulsants

BIOFEEDBACK / PHYSICAL THERAPY

COGNITIVE BEHAVIORAL THERAPY
SEXUAL COUNSELLING

2-3 Months Treatment → Good Relief → Stop Treatment When Indicated

Inadequate /Insufficient Relief

SECOND Therapeutical Step

Multilevel infiltration
-Trigger point steroid and Local Anesthetic injections
-Impar Ganglion sympathetic Block
-Botulinum Toxin

Radiofrequency (RF) procedures
Impar Ganglion abliation
RF sacral rhizotomy thermolesion Sacral nerve roots modulation with pulsedRF

Neurostimulation procedures
Intravaginal transcutaneous electrical nerve stimulation
Spinal cord stimulation
Selective stimulation of sacral nerve roots S2S3S4
Subcutaneous vulvar stimulation

Maintenance of first step
VULVAR CARE MEASURES
BIOFEEDBACK / PHYSICAL THERAPY
COGNITIVE BEHAVIORAL / SEXUAL COUNSELLING

2-3 Months Treatment → Good Relief → Stop Treatment When Indicated

Inadequate/Insufficient Relief

THIRD Therapeutical Step

SURGERY
Local Excision
Vestibulectomy
Perineoplasty
Surgery on Pudendal Nerve Entrapment

Chapter 7

Oral Medication for Vulvodynia

There are many oral medications (medications taken by mouth) you can use to treat vulvodynia. With these medications, the goal is to take the lowest dose possible so you can enjoy maximum relief with minimal side effects. Sometimes, you may need to take a combination of medications to get the best results.

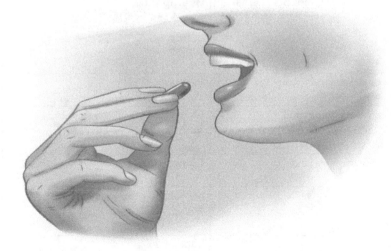

Anti-epileptic medications (AEDs), antidepressants, and other types of medications are often used to treat vulvodynia. Most of these medications were originally created to serve a different purpose, but doctors have found that they're also effective in treating other issues.

For example, pregabalin was created to treat epilepsy, but is now used to treat neuropathic pain and anxiety as well.

Below is a list of oral medications often used to treat vulvodynia, listed by class (or drug type), and name. Other medications are and have been used. Each class interacts with the body in a different way, and different classes can be effective for different people.

Oral Medications Used in the Treatment of Vulvodynia

Medication Class	Medication Name
Anti-epileptic drugs (AEDs)	Carbamazepine Gabapentin Pregabalin Levetiracetam Lamotrigine Oxcarbazepine Topiramate
Tricyclic Antidepressants (TCAs)	Amitriptyline Dosulepin Nortriptyline Imipramine
Selective Serotonin Reuptake Inhibitor (SSRI) Antidepressants	Paroxetine
Selective Serotonin and Norepinephrine Reuptake Inhibitor (SSNRI) Antidepressants	Duloxetine Venlafaxine
Benzodiazepines (BDZ)	Clonazepam
Medicinal Cannabis	See Chapter 8. Medical Cannabis for Vulvodynia
Weak Opioids	Tapentadol Tramadol
Strong Opioids	Morphine Oxycodone

What to Know Before Starting a New Medication

Before starting you on a new medication, your doctor should spend some time talking through your medical history, checking if you're allergic to any drugs, and seeing if you have any health conditions that will conflict with the new medication. They should also make sure you're not currently taking any medications that will interact negatively with the new prescription.

If you're thinking of becoming pregnant or breast feeding, or if you suddenly become pregnant while taking vulvodynia medication, tell your doctor immediately. It's important to make sure the medication you're taking won't carry any negative side effects for you and your child.

Finding the Right Prescription

Because there are so many different treatments for vulvodynia, there's no one medication that's right or wrong to start with. Your doctor will probably recommend one that they've found to be successful, and/or one that will be safe and effective for you.

You'll start with a low dose, then slowly increase until you achieve maximum pain relief with minimal side effects. Usually, if you do experience side effects, you'll notice within the first few days, and your side effects will probably go away with time. If they don't, or if your side effects are especially severe, your doctor may recommend lowering your dose or changing to a different medication. Later, after your system has gotten used to the medication, your doctor may increase the dosage. If you feel like your dose needs to be changed, either because you're not experiencing enough relief, or because you're experiencing negative side effects, talk to your doctor.

Finding the right dosage and combination of medications is often just a matter of trial and error. Sometimes, this process is very easy. You may find that the first medication you try works quickly and carries no side effects. Or, you may have to experiment with multiple medications before you find one, or a combination, that works. Depending on which medications are effective and how you tolerate them, this process can take anywhere from a couple of weeks to several months.

Next Steps

Eventually, you and your doctor should be able to identify the best type, combination, and dosage of medication to treat your pain with minimal side effects. Now, we don't want you to be taking this medication for the rest of your life. Instead, the goal is to keep you on it long enough for your nervous system to heal and start functioning normally, usually around six months. Then, if possible, you'll start slowly weaning off the medication, as advised by your doctor.

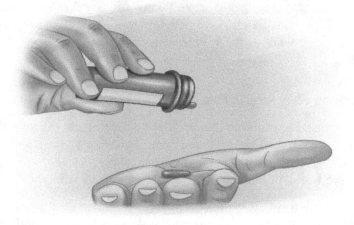

How to Take Vulvodynia Medication Safely

1. Follow the instructions and your doctor's guidance

Always take medication according to the instructions on the package and according to your doctor's advice. Never take medications for longer than your doctor recommends, and never take them in a different quantity [1]. Consult with your doctor before you stop taking a medication, and be mindful of any conditions you have that may interact negatively with the prescription. Remember, it may take several weeks before you notice the medication making a difference.

2. Stick to the schedule and don't overdose

Your doctor may recommend taking doses on a schedule. For example, you may take one in the morning and one at night, or you may simply take one a day. It's easy to forget and miss a dose, but if you do, don't panic. Unless your doctor tells you otherwise, simply take the dose you missed as soon as you remember. If it's almost time for your next scheduled dose, just skip the missed dose and continue taking the medication as scheduled. Don't take extra medication to compensate for the missed dose [1]. If you're not sure what to do, talk to your doctor or pharmacist.

If you do overdose, call for emergency help immediately. Overdose symptoms may include fainting, seizure (convulsions), muscle stiffness, feeling hot or cold, hallucinations, vomiting, confusion, extreme drowsiness, and an uneven heartbeat [1].

3. Watch for side effects

All medications can carry potential negative side effects, but most of these effects only last for a few days. If you experience side effects that are especially severe or that last for more than a few days, talk to your doctor or pharmacist as soon as you can.

Some common side effects include feeling tired, drowsy, sleepy, fatigued, and dizzy. You can learn more about possible side effects on the drug sheets that come with your tablets or capsules. Don't let the list of side effects scare you, though. Manufacturers are legally required to include all possible side effects, but most of these are rare. You're much more likely to experience minor, temporary side effects, or none at all. Still, it's important to be aware.

One reason you may experience side effects is if you're taking another drug that interacts with the new medication. This can happen with prescription and over-the-counter drugs, herbal products, and vitamins. That's why you'll want to tell your doctor about any and all medications and vitamins you're currently taking, and don't start a new medication without talking to your doctor first [1].

If your throat, tongue, lips, or face swell up, or if you get hives or have trouble breathing, you may be having an allergic reaction to your medication [1]. If this happens, seek emergency medical help right away. Again, this is something you probably won't have to worry about, as it's very rare, but it's always good to be prepared.

If you do start to experience side effects, your doctor may recommend splitting the doses throughout the day, taking higher doses in the evening, or taking a different combination of medications.

4. Use alcohol with caution

Combining medication with alcohol can lead to serious side effects, so it's best to use alcohol with caution while on your medication. If, while on the medication, you notice any worrying symptoms that occur with alcohol use, contact your doctor and stop using alcohol until you can talk to them about it.

5. Store your medication securely

Store your medications at room temperature away from light, heat, and moisture [1]. You can usually find more information about storage on the package or drug sheet. Remember to keep your medication out of sight and reach of children.

6. Be careful driving

Some medications can impair your thinking and reactions, so be careful driving or doing anything else that requires a high level of alertness or quick reactions, like operating machinery or tools [1]. Talk to your doctor if you're concerned about this.

7. Protect your skin

Some medications can make your skin more sensitive to light. Your doctor should tell you if this is the case, and if it is, be sure to use sun lotion with an SPF (sun protection factor) of 30 or higher. It's also a good idea to wear protective clothing when you're out in the sun [1].

Is Anti-Epileptic Medication Addictive?

Gabapentin (GBP), pregabalin (PG), and other anti-epileptic drugs prescribed for nerve pain are largely misunderstood, which is why they're not often prescribed for vulvodynia. Some general practitioners are resistant to prescribing them, and many patients worry that they will become addicted. But it's worth noting that, unlike opioids, GBP and PG are not addictive. When taken under the guidance of a qualified doctor, this type of medication is generally very safe. If your doctor is reluctant to prescribe you this medication, seek support from your pain specialist or primary care physician, depending on the situation.

Recap of Oral Medication for Vulvodynia

- Follow your doctor's guidance when taking medications.

- When starting a new medication, take small doses first and increase slowly until you achieve maximum pain relief with minimal side effects.

- Most side effects are minor and only last for a few days.

- Once you find a dosage or combination that works, continue taking it for a finite period, usually around six months, then start to reduce the dosage according to your doctor's instructions.

- The goal is to treat your pain and then get you off the medication, so you're not taking it for any longer than you need to be.

- Take medication safely by following the package instructions, talking to your doctor about any possible complications, watching for side effects, and taking your doses as scheduled.

Sources of Information on Medications

British National Formulary

https://bnf.nice.org.uk/

Drugs.com

https://www.drugs.com/

Summary of Product Characteristics (SPC or SmPC)

This document describes the properties and officially approved usage of a medication. Healthcare professionals use summaries of product characteristics as a basis for using medicine safely and effectively. You can find these easily online.

PubMed

PubMed contains more than 30 million citations for biomedical literature from MEDLINE, life science journals, and online books. Citations may include links to full-text content from PubMed Central and publisher websites.

https://pubmed.ncbi.nlm.nih.gov/

"Success rates in studies of pharmacologic interventions for vestibulodynia vary from no effect to 100%" [2].

For further information on specific medications, please see the following at the end of the book:

Appendix A. Popular Oral Medications Which Can be Prescribed for Vulvodynia

Chapter 8

Topical Medication for Vulvodynia

Nathaniel Jones, R.Ph, FAPC

Disclaimer: Nathaniel Jones is an employee of PCCA—a company that provides education, research, and materials for the creation of bespoke medications—and as such, his perspective may reflect his industry's financial interests.

We've now discussed different aspects of vulvodynia and some of the treatments available. In this chapter, we'll review a different option, topical treatments.

The idea of applying pain medication to a painful place is a simple one, and can help not only by treating pain symptoms, but by helping to treat the underlying condition itself. The big advantage of a topical treatment, as opposed to an oral one, is that since you don't take it orally, it does not enter the gastrointestinal tract. This decreases the likelihood of potential negative side effects and drug-to-drug interactions.

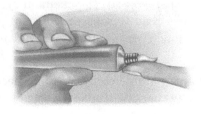

You can also potentially get higher levels of the medication right to the area where you need it most. In general, when you take a medication by mouth, it gets distributed throughout the entire body with only a very small portion reaching the site where you need it to go. So, in order to get enough medication where you need it, you end up taking a lot more.

But by applying it topically, you are targeting the medication to the area where the pain is located, and so you can usually use less. This is beneficial because medications must be metabolized and eliminated, so less medication in means less medication liability to deal with overall. Potentially, this can make topical applications safer than oral use at higher doses.

Another interesting point about topical treatment is that multiple medication combinations can be applied in the same formulation. In other words, instead of applying multiple medications, you'll only need to apply one. And since you're applying medication to a small and sensitive area, the less the better. Combining multiple active pharmaceutical ingredients in a single topical dose can increase the probability of a successful outcome, especially if the pain is multifaceted and requires different drug therapies simultaneously.

Neuropathy

The word "neuro" refers to the nerves or nervous system. Neuropathy is damage, disease, or dysfunction of one or more nerves, especially of the peripheral nervous system. (The peripheral nervous system includes all the nerves outside the brain and spinal cord.) The pain associated with this phenomenon is called neuropathic pain (nerve pain). Neuropathic pain often feels like a shooting, stabbing, burning, numbness, or tingling.

Vulvodynia pain is neuropathic, which means it's likely caused by abnormal signals from the nerves in the vulvar area. These nerve endings are hypersensitive, so the pain may be constant or intermittent. As we've already discussed, constant pain that happens when there is no touch or pressure is known as unprovoked vulvodynia.

When neuropathic pain occurs, it may be because the nervous system inappropriately changes or adapts. Instead of sending a simple one-off pain message to the brain, the nervous system becomes locked on, continually sending the message. It may start with a simple acute pain message from inflammation, infection, or trauma that would normally go away as the injury heals. But for some unknown reason, the pain messaging system becomes locked on, causing you to develop chronic neuropathic pain. Learning how to break this vicious cycle of events can be key to overcoming vulvodynia.

Imagine the nervous system as electrical wiring. Sometimes neuropathic pain is not triggered just at the location where you feel the pain, but further back in the wiring. As is the case with so many electrically controlled devices, the actual problem may be located at a relay switch or in the central computer.

For example, many patients have problems in their spinal column, and this causes pain in their legs and feet. While they experience pain in their extremities, the real location that needs treatment is their back. So, believe it or not, application of topical treatments to the back may improve vulvodynia pain for some women. Back therapy taken along with a topical vulvar application may also help the pain. In any case, the site of application on the back is important, because the medication needs to be applied to the area beside the vertebrae. This is the area through which the nerves that feed into the genital region originate.

The type of topical medication is also important. The skin on the back, like most of the body, has an outer layer of protection, and this layer can be resistant to certain kinds of drug delivery. So, if you're applying medication to the back, that medication needs to have a topical delivery base that permeates the skin, allowing it to reach the spinal column. These bases are known as transdermal delivery bases, or permeation enhanced topical delivery bases.

When applying topical medication, keep in mind the following:

- Part of the skin covering the outer labia acts as a protective barrier. This can affect a drug's ability to penetrate into the tissue underneath.

- The inner labia does not have this protective barrier, so it's much easier for medication to penetrate there. This is also true of the opening, or introitus, and interior of the vagina.

- When you apply medication to the inner labia, though the tissue can be more delicate and sensitive, your body will absorb the medication more completely and more rapidly. That makes the inner labia a good place to apply medication to.

Old Medications, New Uses

Several topical medications are used to treat vulvodynia, but these drugs are considered unlicensed for this use, which means they need to be prescribed by a doctor and manufactured by a licensed facility. Specialists are still studying the effectiveness of these medications in treating vulvodynia.

However, while they may not be officially licensed to treat vulvodynia, these drug ingredients are well-known to medical practitioners, and doctors have been prescribing them to treat other conditions for decades now. So rather than thinking of these as new drugs, think of them as old drugs being used in a new way.

Some people are concerned when they learn that these drugs are unlicensed for vulvodynia. But unlicensed prescribing is perfectly legal in the US, Canada, UK, and Australia. Many practitioners routinely prescribe drugs for unlicensed use, especially in pediatrics, psychiatry, and palliative care—often because unlicensed drugs are necessary to meet the specific needs of their patients.

Of course, in a perfect world, we would have study data supporting the use of every aspect of every drug for all types of patients and every disease. Since we don't live in a perfect world, that level of utopian medicine is unlikely to ever be achieved. Meanwhile, as long as people have problems that can't be solved in the traditional ways, unlicensed prescribing remains a reasonable option.

Next, we will review the five main topical medications that practitioners have studied in the treatment of vulvodynia. We'll also briefly look at the level of proof or evidence for how well each of these medications work. The five drugs are: gabapentin, lidocaine, amitriptyline, baclofen, and capsaicin.

Topical Gabapentin

Gabapentin (brand name Neurontin) was approved in 1993 for the treatment of partial seizures with and without secondary generalization. Years later, it was approved for peripheral neuropathic pain, including painful diabetic neuropathy and post-herpetic neuralgia.

The oral tablets and capsules have a long track record of treating neuropathic pain, so it's no surprise doctors have studied it as a topical treatment for vulvodynia. According to the NHS, gabapentin has been reclassified as a controlled medicine under the Misuse of Drugs Act 1971 (from April 1, 2019). Interestingly, the potential for abuse of gabapentin in a topical preparation is considered extremely low due to poor topical permeation.

In 2008, researchers conducted a study with topical gabapentin on 51 women with chronic vulvodynia. 22 of the women used 6% gabapentin cream, 19 used 2%, and 11 used 4%. At the end of the study, 80% of the women demonstrated at least a 50% improvement in pain scores, and 29% reported complete pain relief. Among those with localized vulvodynia, sexual function improved in 17 of 20 women [1]. While oral gabapentin tends to bring negative side effects, none of the women taking it topically reported any of these side effects. Overall, the medication was very well tolerated. 7 out of 51 women discontinued the cream due to local irritation, but it's unclear if this irritation was caused by the gabapentin itself or by the base used to prepare the cream. This may simply indicate how important it is to choose the right cream base for the application location.

As discussed in this study, gabapentin is usually applied topically for vulvodynia in strengths ranging from 2% up to 6%. A 6% topical cream will provide 60mg of gabapentin per gram of cream. Oral dosages of gabapentin, for fibromyalgia for example, usually start at 300mg orally three times per day and can go up to 3,600mg per day. Side effects from large oral dosages include drowsiness, dizziness, physical weakness, ataxia (slurred speech, stumbling, falling, and incoordination), and headache. But as mentioned above, these side events were not reported by any of the women in the study, and overall, treatment was very well tolerated.

Topical Lidocaine

One drug that's been around for a long time is lidocaine, also known as lignocaine, a local anesthetic drug used to numb tissues. Many women have tried using it to treat vulvodynia, but no one has done a well-designed, long-term study to evaluate its performance. In the last decade, researchers have done a few small studies, but the results were not as favorable as was hoped for.

One study used topical lidocaine with an oral antidepressant medication (Desipramine). Although the medication was well-tolerated, it was not effective [2]. However, lidocaine has been shown to treat other types of neuropathic pain, so it stands to reason that it could be useful for vulvodynia, perhaps in a better designed topical formulation or as part of a comprehensive treatment plan [2].

Lidocaine is usually applied topically for vulvodynia by itself or in combinations, from a 1% to 5% cream or gel in a gentle base suitable for vaginal/vulvar application. As with most medications, the less the better. The smallest dosage amount that does the job is the right amount to use.

Topical Amitriptyline

Amitriptyline, an antidepressant, has long been used orally in the treatment of neuropathic pain. Some studies have shown that topical amitriptyline helps with painful intercourse (dyspareunia), a common symptom of vulvodynia [3].

Amitriptyline is usually applied topically in a strength of 2% to 5% for vulvodynia. While one study had patients use a 10% cream, that may be too strong for some women. The safety mantra is to start low and go slow, so it's best to gradually increase after trying the lowest strength first.

Topical Baclofen

Baclofen was originally approved in 1977 for use as an oral skeletal muscle relaxant (primarily for spasticity) and was later found to be useful in treating neuropathic pain [4].

One case study tested topical baclofen 5% cream with oral palmitoylethanolamide, a drug used to treat neuropathic pain. After one month, the woman using baclofen reported that her pain decreased by about 30%. After three months, she was able to have undisturbed sexual intercourse, sit for hours, and ride a bicycle. Her pain decreased on a ten-point scale from 6-7 down to 2, with periods of no pain at all [5].

Obviously, one successful case study does not mean this solution will work for all vulvodynia sufferers. As researchers are notorious for saying, "further research is needed" before we can seriously recommend treatment. But it is evidence, albeit far from conclusive. After all, individual case studies are usually how medical research gets started.

Baclofen is commonly used topically for vulvodynia pain at 2%, often in combination with one or more of the five medications discussed here, but as this case study mentions, up to 5% is possible. It is usually formulated in a cream base that is safe for vaginal use, or in a muco-adhesive gel base if applied to the mucous membranes of the vagina or inner labia. The latter allows for longer contact time.

Topical Capsaicin

The chemical capsaicin was first isolated from chili peppers in crystalline form in the late 1800s. Considered a chemical irritant, it produces a burning sensation in the tissue with which it comes into contact, including mucous membranes.

If it causes burning, you may be asking, why use it to treat vulvodynia? Isn't this condition already painful enough?

Yes, but by stimulating the nerve endings in the tissues, capsaicin ultimately reduces pain signals. While it may burn at first, the outcome may be well worth it if the treatment is successful.

Capsaicin is currently used in topical form for neuropathic pain like postherpetic neuralgia (shingles pain) and diabetic neuropathy, and to relieve painful skin conditions like osteo, rheumatoid, and psoriatic arthritis. One study using capsaicin 0.025% cream for vulvar vestibulitis syndrome showed that it significantly decreases discomfort and allows for more frequent sexual relations [6].

One downside is that the strength of capsaicin needs to be increased over time to maintain the same level of pain control. But on the upside, applying a numbing agent like lidocaine prior to capsaicin use can reduce or eliminate the initial burning sensation.

More Options for Relief

There are more drugs that may be useful, but which have yet to be studied in clinical vulvodynia trials. These include ketamine, naltrexone, and cannabidiol.

Topical Ketamine

Ketamine, a drug that got its start in the sixties for surgical anesthesia, has more recently been used in permeation enhanced topical delivery bases to treat various forms of neuropathic pain. While no studies have been done on using this drug to treat vulvodynia, some doctors have reported that topical ketamine in low percentage concentrations works for their patients.

Topical Naltrexone

Naltrexone has been available for decades, primarily to help opioid-dependent patients stay drug-free. It's also been used to treat a variety of conditions, including some dermatologic conditions and pain. A growing number of practitioners report success using topical naltrexone 0.5% to treat vulvodynia.

The idea of taking oral low dose naltrexone (0.5mg up to 5mg daily at bedtime), or LDN, began in the eighties to help improve the immune systems of patients with AIDS. Although lacking large clinical studies, LDN has gained popularity for treating a large variety of diseases, including many autoimmune diseases, and has been the subject of a number of smaller studies. Some of those studies have shown potential for using LDN to treat Crohn's disease, Multiple Sclerosis, pain (including Fibromyalgia and Complex Regional Pain Syndrome), and skin diseases (including Pemphigus and Psoriasis).

LDN may also help treat the pain and depressive symptoms that often accompany vulvodynia.

Topical Medicinal Cannabis

Cannabidiol, or CBD, is one of the major components in medicinal cannabis, which may be effective for treating neuropathic and inflammatory pain. In fact, numerous preclinical studies have shown that medicinal cannabis can help with pelvic pain. As of the date of this publication, no one has conducted a clinical trial for using CBD to treat vulvodynia. But since neuropathy and inflammation are associated with vulvodynia, it seems likely that these studies will be conducted soon.

If you're uncomfortable with the idea of taking medicinal cannabis, know that some forms of CBD can be made from citrus limonene instead of from hemp, and that the type of CBD used to treat neuropathic pain is free from THC, the psychoactive component of cannabis. Many manufacturers in the UK make this non-psychoactive form of CBD.

We'll discuss CBD in more detail in the next chapter.

Questions about Topical Medications for Vulvodynia

If you and your practitioner decide to try one of these topical formulations for your vulvodynia, what can you expect to happen?

Women who decide to try a topical medication often ask questions like: How long will it take before this works? Will this be a cure or an ongoing treatment? Is it safe to use before having sex or should I worry about my partner being exposed? How long after I use this do I need to wait before engaging in sexual activity? What side effects will I have, if any? Is it safe?

Because large-scale, randomized clinical trials have not been conducted for most of these medications due to a lack of funding, the answers to these questions mainly come from anecdotal reports, based on the experiences of other women who's used these formulations. Let's take these questions one at a time.

How long will it take before this works?

How long it takes for a topical treatment to work varies from drug to drug, so there is no one-size-fits-all answer to this question. Local anesthetics like lidocaine usually work in less than 45 minutes, but the effects may only last for a couple of hours. Whereas gabapentin can take over a week to start working, the effects may last 4 to 6 hours after each application. Ask your doctor for more specific information about the medication you are taking.

Is this a cure or an ongoing treatment?

This will likely be a symptomatic treatment. Your condition may go into remission for months to years, though it's more common for vulvodynia to persist. The point of topical medication may be to help lessen your symptoms while you and your practitioner try to find a more permanent solution.

Is it safe to use before having sex or should I worry about my partner being exposed?

If possible, it's best not to apply the medication directly before sexual activity. Although these drugs are reasonably well-tolerated and there's no reason to expect your partner would have a negative response, there's no need to expose someone else to potentially negative effects.

How long after I use this do I need to wait before engaging in sexual activity?

That depends on the base of delivery for the topical, but a safe estimate would be about 24 hours. If your partner is sensitive to the medication, it may be best to wait longer. Ask your doctor for more specific information about the formulation you are using.

What side effects will I have, if any?

There's a possibility that you'll develop local irritation from the treatment. This could be due in part to one of the drugs, or it could simply be due to an individual intolerance to the topical base used. Topical bases quite often contain 10 or more ingredients, so there's a chance you may develop sensitivity to one or more of them. If this happens, consult your doctor.

Is it safe?

As mentioned, these drugs have been around for decades. When dosed properly, they are quite safe. In fact, a topical application may be safer than an oral one, as it decreases the amount of drug absorbed. Because of this, the odds of experiencing a significant safety issue are very low.

When taken orally, some of these drugs, like gabapentin and amitriptyline, can cause drowsiness. But when applied topically, they rarely do. That's because, as we've discussed already, when a drug is taken by mouth, it enters the blood stream at a higher concentration, and more of it gets to the brain, allowing for side effects like drowsiness. By taking medication topically, you can bypass this issue.

Using Topical Medications for Your Treatment

Your doctor will likely choose a formulation for you based on details like the nature of your condition, your pain level, and your sensitivity to certain ingredients. Choosing which set of ingredients to include is a process that's unique to each patient, as is choosing the cream or gel base for topical delivery. Since not everyone tolerates the same products equally, there are many different base options. Some patients are sensitive to certain ingredients and require a special topical base to avoid the offending ingredient. If this is the case, there's usually a drug manufacturer who can accommodate the request, but it may take a little longer to get approval for the needed formula.

As you begin topical treatment for your vulvodynia, it can be easy to lose patience. Just remember that you did not develop vulvodynia overnight, and you are not likely to get relief overnight either. Rather than looking for a miracle cure, start with slow, steady progress and work from there. Most of the time, topical medications are just one part of a multifaceted approach to treating vulvodynia. "An individualized, holistic, and often multidisciplinary approach is needed to effectively manage the patient's pain and pain-related distress" [7].

It may be helpful to keep in mind the following about vulvodynia treatment:

- It's not an exact science.

- It's still a trial-and-error process.

- It usually does not provide instantaneous relief.

- Since no two patients are the same, treatment should be customized to fit the individual on a case-by-case basis.

- Since there's rarely a single, fix-all solution for vulvodynia, you're most likely to find relief through a combination of treatments.

Bespoke topical treatment combinations may be more beneficial than single drug therapies, as they offer multiple mechanisms of action, which may increase success. It's less likely for a single drug therapy to work for everyone, but combinations can cast a wider net. Critics may say that if multiple ingredients are used, it's unclear what's working and what's not. But if all the individual ingredients have shown some success in the past for other women, albeit not all women, there's a higher possibility of a positive outcome.

Getting Started

As part of an overall treatment plan, topical drug therapy for vulvodynia offers pain relief and hope for many women.

So how do you get started with a topical treatment? Simply ask your doctor or clinician if they're willing to prescribe a formula that might offer you some relief. It may be wise to consult with a gynecologist or pain physician who's familiar with such treatments, or have your practitioner consult with one on your behalf.

Chapter 9

Medical Cannabis for Vulvodynia

The Body's Endocannabinoid System

It may surprise you to learn that the body naturally produces its own cannabinoids, called endocannabinoids, that help keep the body's internal physical and chemical conditions steady. These endocannabinoids are involved in virtually every one of the body's systems, including the nervous system, lungs, digestive system, liver, spleen, and many of the body's circulating blood cells. Endocannabinoids are produced from eicosanoids, local hormonal molecules that also go into the make-up of many other molecules affecting different body systems.

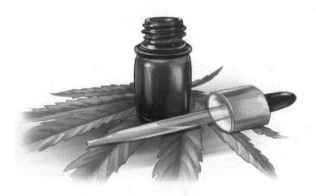

There are three basic receptors (molecules that respond specifically to a certain stimulus) for cannabis molecules in the body:

- CB1 which binds to Anandamide (the body's equivalent of THC)

- CB2 which binds to 2-AG (2-arachidonolglycerol), the body's equivalent of Cannabidiol

- CB3 which increases intracellular calcium to keep the body functioning normally, and which responds to many of the different cannabinoid molecules.

The endocannabinoid system affects many of the body's functions, including:

- appetite and digestion

- metabolism

- chronic pain

- inflammation and other immune system responses

- mood

- learning and memory

- motor control

- sleep

- cardiovascular system function

- muscle formation

- bone remodeling and growth

- liver function

- reproductive system function

- stress

- skin and nerve function

Since its re-introduction as a medicine that can be prescribed in many countries, research into the endocannabinoid system is rapidly increasing, and we're starting to discover more about how this complex system manages many of the body's systems.

Consequently, specialist cannabis medicine clinics are starting to recognize the immense benefits of cannabis for treating complex diseases., including conditions where pain is a major symptom.

Let's briefly discuss some of the current uses of medicinal cannabis and look at how they may help you with vulvodynia. First, we'll review the basics about medical cannabis.

Cannabinoids: CBD and THC

Cannabinoids are chemicals found naturally in the cannabis plant. One of the most common of these is cannabidiol (CBD). Directly derived from hemp, CBD is a cousin of the marijuana plant. Another common chemical is tetrahydrocannabinol (THC), an abundant natural compound with a higher content in the marijuana plant. THC is the main psychoactive compound that gives many marijuana users the "high sensation" [5].

Cannabidiol (CBD) is one of over a hundred cannabinoid compounds in the cannabis plant, all of which have different actions. In addition to the Terpenes (which give it its characteristic smell), and flavoproteins, there are some 500 different molecules in the cannabis plant. CBD does not generate a high by itself.

Even the active THC (tetrahydrocannabinol), which is what gives users the psychological high, must be heated to do so (hence why it's often smoked or cooked). As the WHO has stated "In humans, CBD exhibits no effects indicative of any abuse or dependence potential.... to date, there is no evidence of public health related problems associated with the use of pure CBD" [1]. None of the cannabis molecules are physically addictive, since there are no changes in the body (as occurs with opioids, for example). Over 65% of patients seeking cannabis medications do so to help treat pain, not to "get high."

You may be in a country or state where you can easily obtain medical cannabis (medical marijuana), but if this approach does not appeal to you, or if you cannot obtain it, there is an alternative. This is cannabidiol, or CBD, which is derived from hemp and is readily available in many countries in forms like gels, oils, extracts, and more.

"Pain-reduction is one of the most common therapeutic uses for cannabinoids" [2].

The Lowdown on Relieving Pain with CBD and THC

While cannabidiol (CBD) does not have the same psychoactive level as THC (tetrahydrocannabinol, which is the chemical responsible for most of marijuana's psychological effects), it's been known to "positively influence mood, and can help manage the dysphoria associated with pain. Additionally, CBD can boost opioid-based analgesic effects, enabling patients to achieve efficacy (benefit) with lower doses of opioids, reducing the risk of addiction and overdose" [3,6].

While THC delivers the euphoric and psychoactive high of cannabis, a large percentage of people would like to use it minus these side effects. Fortunately, "small amounts of THC can provide pain relief, reduce inflammation, and relax muscles, without producing powerful psychoactive effects" [3]. In other words, women may not have to experience psychoactivity if they want to treat their vulvodynia using THC [3].

Taken together, CBD and THC work in harmony to provide a more powerful effect than either can produce on their own. Broad spectrum cannabis medicine products (which include all the molecules from the cannabis plant) with defined amounts of CBD and THC are generally more effective than individual isolates of CBD or THC. This is known as the 'entourage' effect. It simply means that all the molecules of cannabis are working together.

In the entourage effect, all the cannabis molecules contained in the oils extracted from the cannabis plant work in different ways to relieve different aspects of illness. In addition to the known cannabis molecules contained in cannabis oil, the terpenes, a combination of molecules that give cannabis its characteristic smell, can also affect certain receptors in the nervous and other systems, improving mood and helping wakefulness or sleepiness.

One of the molecules released by metabolism of THC has anti-inflammatory effects 26 times more potent than any drug currently available. The more we learn about the endocannabinoid system, the more we discover how much the body's cannabinoids may be lacking, and hence, why they respond so well to medicinal cannabis.

"The endocannabinoid system (biological system in the human body that is made up of cannabinoid receptors) has been shown to balance the body, and cannabinoids such as CBD and THC can help" [3].

Other Cannabinoid Chemicals

Tetrahydrocannabinolic acid (THCa)

THCa (tetrahydrocannabinolic acid) is a non-psychoactive, non-impairing cannabinoid. Due to its structure, THCa does not induce a "high." When used medicinally, THCa may help relieve mild pain and inflammation. Some studies have shown that "THCa is more water-soluble than THC, so patients can use lower doses to achieve relief, which reduces cost and adverse side effects" [3].

THCa is the precursor of THC. If you're using THCa for medical relief, be sure to store it in a cool, dark place. This prevents it from being exposed to prolonged UV light and heat, which will convert the THCa to THC and therefore generate psychoactivity [3].

Cannabidiolic acid (CBDa)

"Some conditions, like chronic pain, have a large body of scientific evidence in favor of phytocannabinoid supplementation" [2].

CBDa (cannabidiolic acid) is another non-psychoactive cannabinoid helpful for relieving inflammation. While CBDa has not been studied as much as THC or CBD, "observational reports suggest that CBDa helps with mild pain and fatigue" [3]. Like THCa, CBDa is "more water-soluble than CBD, so patients can use lower doses of CBDa to achieve relief, which reduces cost and adverse side effects" [3].

CBDa is the precursor of CBD. Again like THCa, CBDa must be stored in a cool, dark place to prevent it from being exposed to prolonged UV light and heat, which will convert it to CBD [3].

Cannabigerol (CBG)

As the cannabis plant matures, cannabigerolic acid (CBGa) becomes THCa and CBDa, along with another precursor called CBCA (cannabichromenic acid). Any amounts of CBGa not converted into these precursors then become minor cannabinoids such as CBG.

Like THCa and CBDa, CBG (cannabigerol) is an anti-inflammatory, non-psychoactive cannabinoid. It can "inhibit the uptake of the neurotransmitter GABA, which can decrease anxiety and muscle tension. Further, CBG might offer therapeutic potential as an antidepressant, and as an analgesic" [3].

The Endocannabinoid System and Estrogen

The hormone estrogen can help lower depression and anxiety in women. Recent studies show that estrogen produces these emotionally stabilizing effects because it interacts with the endocannabinoid system. When women go through menopause, their endocannabinoids increase while their estrogen decreases. Lower estrogen also decreases vaginal secretions and increases pain. "Phytocannabinoids [or cannabinoids that occur naturally in the cannabis plant] can be used to counterbalance this increased sensitivity" [2].

It's normal to experience changes and fluctuations within the endocannabinoid system. But this fluctuation won't be the same for everyone, and a percentage of women experience systematically higher or lower levels of endocannabinoids. When the endocannabinoid system is out of balance, various disorders and diseases can follow. Painful sex is one possible result.

Unfortunately, like many areas of cannabinoids, we lack definitive studies on this subject. As Moore remarks, "Clinical trials for different cannabis therapeutics are currently underway, but the medical field is still years away from providing actionable advice for many of these imbalances" [2].

Even so, there is significant evidence available for using cannabinoid products to relieve pain, and as such, it's certainly worthwhile to try some of the methods mentioned in this chapter.

While studies are not yet fully conclusive in this field, we can make some reasonable observations based on estrogen studies. Estrogen is like phytocannabinoids in both fat-solubility and size. For example, when women opt to take estrogen via their vagina, their reproductive tissues receive higher concentrations.

"Based on reports from women who use cannabinoid preparations, when applied inside the vagina, near the cervix, some preparations deliver cannabinoids to the muscles and tissue of the uterus and vagina" [2]. Alternately, cannabinoid arousal oils are another option which work on the vagina and vulva [2].

Delivery Methods

Once you've pinpointed the cannabinoids that may work best for your situation, you'll want to consider the delivery method, specifically, the benefits you'll gain from each method [3]. Ask your doctor or other healthcare professional for help understanding the different formulations and delivery methods. They can also help you learn which forms of cannabinoids are available in your country.

Topical Administration

Topical CBD, which penetrates the top layers of the skin, can offer local pain relief. This relief may act immediately and last for a few hours. "Studies suggest that CBD penetrates the skin more effectively than THC" [3], so a CBD-dominant topical is probably the best way to go.

Keep in mind that your experience taking cannabinoids via your vagina will vary from that of other women, based on factors like your age, where you are in your menstrual cycle, and the thickness of your outer layer of skin [2].

Ingestion

Ingestion (oral intake) can offer systemic relief that may last longer than other methods, and can, over time, reduce inflammation. "Patients report that, when they use cannabis regularly and consistently, they can reduce the severity and intensity of their symptoms" [3]. Over time, it may be possible to lower your overall cannabis intake without losing any of the benefits.

It's important to note however, that edible products (such as baked goods), can generate intense full-body, psychoactive effects, and to that end, they are not recommended.

Sublingual Administration

Sublingual refers to the medication being placed under the tongue. If you are interested in this option, make sure to purchase an authentic sublingual product (one that has a cannabinoid formulation which is more water-soluble than normal). This should take effect within 15 minutes, as the tissues in the mouth quickly absorb the medication [3].

Transdermal Administration

Transdermal products are like topical creams. However, to enable cannabinoids to penetrate the skin and reach the bloodstream, thereby avoiding first-pass metabolism, an extra agent is added. Transdermal patches may offer pain relief for between eight to twelve hours and may be more reliable and consistent than edible products. Time-released long-lasting patches are often a good option for anyone who has an issue with medication compliance [3].

Inhalation

If your pain is constant or fluctuates in intensity, inhalation may be the best means of managing it. Inhaling can relieve pain quickly and give you maximum control over the dose [3].

Cannabinoid Suppositories

A suppository is an alternative method of delivering a drug. A small, round or cone-shaped object is inserted into the body, usually through the bottom or vagina, then dissolves, releasing its medication inside the body. Cannabinoid suppositories are suppositories that contain cannabinoid products and are designed to bring pain relief.

Moore observes that "The first time they try cannabinoid suppositories, many women are shocked at how effective they are. Cannabinoids address pain in two ways. Not only do they desensitize pain-perceiving nerves, but they also limit inflammation, which is often a major contributor to pain" [3].

So how do cannabinoid suppositories work? Well, cannabidiol (CBD) uses the same enzyme that Ibuprofen does. It diminishes painful cramps by reducing the number of inflammatory prostaglandins, a group of chemicals with variable hormone-like effects, produced by the body [2].

Seek Professional Advice about Which Method to Use

To effectively manage your vulvodynia pain, you may need to use multiple delivery methods. For instance, if your pain is chronic, you may have to apply a topical to your skin, ingest CBD/cannabis throughout the day to relieve the pain, and inhale CBD/cannabis when you experience breakthrough pain.

This decision should be left to an experienced doctor or healthcare practitioner. They can create a plan for you complete with information about frequency and dosing [3].

FAQs about Cannabinoids

Which Dosage Size is Effective?

Because CBD is generally available as an unregulated supplement, and because there is a lack of high-quality studies on CBD usage in humans, pinpointing effective doses is not easy. If you are interested in trying it out, first consult your doctor or experienced cannabis healthcare professional to make sure that you do not have any contraindications (conditions that could interact negatively with the medication), and that using CBD will not interfere with any other medication you are taking. Always read the manufacturer's instructions [1].

Are there Cannabinoid Receptors in the Vulva?

There are cannabinoid receptors spread throughout the female reproductive tract. The uterus contains the highest density of these receptors, but they're also present in the vulva, vagina, ovaries, and fallopian tubes.

As Yale-educated biologist Genevieve Moore notes "on a microscopic level, endocannabinoid receptors are located where they can exert control. They are associated with nerves where they mediate sensations, immune cells where they control inflammation, glands where they influence hormone secretion and muscles where they facilitate energy usage" [2].

Can Cannabinoids Give You Sexual Pleasure?

Some people report being able to get "in the mood" after consuming cannabis. But "this aphrodisiac quality is not just a side-effect of the relaxation and mental 'high.' A growing number of women are applying cannabinoids directly to their vulvas to increase sexual pleasure typically without any noticeable mental effects" [2].

In other words, while some people have found cannabinoids helpful for increasing sexual pleasure, there's little scientific evidence.

Can Phytocannabinoids Help Sexual Arousal?

During sexual arousal, blood engorges the vagina and clitoris, producing lubrication, elongation, and opening. When women apply phytocannabinoids (cannabinoids that occur naturally in the cannabis plant) to their vulva, it generates a similar effect: vasodilation, or dilatation of blood vessels, increases blood flow. At a microscopic level "THC stimulates the release of neurotransmitters, particularly nitric oxide (NO). Nitric oxide causes the smooth muscle of blood vessels to relax, and the blood vessels dilate and swell with blood" [2].

Although we don't yet have enough clinical research to prove this theory, it's possible that hemp-derived CBD stimulates the genitals. While cannabidiol cannot stimulate cannabinoid receptors, it could have an effect on other receptors in the genital region [2].

Will a "High Vagina" Make Me High as Well?

Normally, applying phytocannabinoids via your vagina will not give you a "high." Topical cannabinoids tend to remain in the area where they are applied, and if any get into the bloodstream, they are processed in a different way than vapor or cannabis edibles. This is because they are not processed via the liver, and so do not go through the first-pass metabolism that changes THC into 1-hydroxy-THC, a molecule that produces even greater psychoactive effects [2]. So no, applying cannabinoids to your vagina will not make you high.

Is Medical Cannabis Legal?

In the US, medical cannabis is legal in most states. Two products licensed in the UK are Sativex and Nabilone.

Is CBD Legal?

Hemp-derived CBD (cannabidiol) is easy to purchase in the US and the UK. Five years ago, the FDA made it easier for scientists to carry out cannabidiol trials [1], which was a giant leap forward. At the present time, hemp-derived CBD can be ordered online or purchased in certain shops by US and UK. residents.

What Does the Evidence Say about Chronic Pain?

Cannabidiol (CBD) may well be a useful option for treating various types of long-term pain, including vulvodynia. Peter Grinspoon, MD, of Harvard Medical School, notes "A study from the European Journal of Pain shows that CBD applied on the skin [of animals] could help lower pain and inflammation. Another study demonstrated the mechanism by which CBD inhibits inflammatory and neuropathic pain, two of the most difficult types of chronic pain to treat" [1]. More research into the potential link between CBD and pain control using human subjects is needed.

Is CBD Safe to Use?

While the potential negative effects of CBD number less than those of conventional medications, they do exist. These side effects include irritability, fatigue, and nausea. Cannabidiol can also increase the blood thinner coumadin within the bloodstream, along with various other medications within the bloodstream. It does this using the same mechanism as grapefruit juice [1]. A study showed side effects of inhaled cannabinoids to be sore throat, cough, bad taste, and vomiting, but all these symptoms were rated as mild [7].

One important safety concern is that CBD is not currently considered a medication, but chiefly sold and marketed as a supplement. As the purity and safety of dietary supplements are not currently regulated in the US or UK, there is no guarantee that CBD products contain the active ingredients, or the dose shown on the label. For this reason, you should only purchase CBD from a reputable company [1].

Chapter 10

Pelvic Floor Muscles and Physiotherapy for Vulvodynia

"For many women, the pelvic floor does not work as well as it should. Almost one-quarter of women have pelvic floor disorders, according to a study funded by the National Institutes of Health" [1].

If you have vulvodynia, you may also have pelvic floor muscle dysfunction (PFMD). Tense, shortened, painful pelvic floor muscles (PFM) are referred to as overactive. Alternately, if you are experiencing vulvar pain, you may have vaginismus, a spasm in your PFM. Either way, physiotherapy can help.

When you visit a PFM physiotherapist, they will explain that a combined approach of treatments is often the most successful way forward. These physiotherapists help women with vulvodynia and overactive PFM manage PFMD in a very functional way by focusing on the entire use of the pelvic floor. They take a holistic perspective regarding its ability to contract, lengthen, relax, and strengthen.

"Studies indicate significant clinical effects of physiotherapy for chronic pelvic pain (CPP) and female sexual dysfunction (FSD), and experts advocate a multidisciplinary approach that includes physiotherapy" [2].

Exercises that facilitate PFM lengthening, stretching, and relaxation are known as down-training approaches. Once your PFM have achieved full length and you are pain free, your therapist may recommend up-training, exercises to strengthen the PFM, often used for incontinence. But this probably won't come until later, if at all.

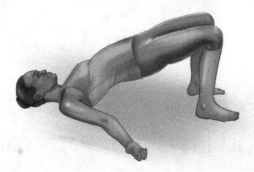

"**Exercising the muscles of the pelvic floor can help strengthen the pelvic floor, and will also help you learn how to relax these muscles when you need to**" [3].

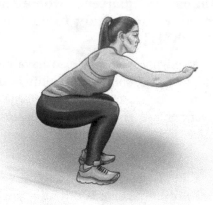

Basic Anatomy

As you seek to understand how your PFM work, it's helpful to know some basic anatomy [3]. If you don't understand all the technical terms in this section, don't worry. They're simply there for reference. The most important thing to understand is not to compartmentalise the pelvic floor too much. In fact, when teaching anatomy to patients, physiotherapists encourage them to think about using the pelvic floor functionally as a whole unit. In other words, try to imagine every muscle in your pelvic floor working together in unison.

The PFM span the bottom of the pelvis and support the pelvic organs including bladder, bowel, and uterus. Weak PFM can lead to problems with bladder and bowel control.

The pelvic floor is comprised of three main muscle layers:

- **Layer 1.** Known as the superficial group, this set of muscles is found at the vagina entrance. The muscles in the superficial group help with bladder control and sexual function; but events such as childbirth, excessive heavy lifting, chronic constipation, peri-menopause, menopause, and aging can cause these muscles to weaken [3]. The muscles include: bulbocavernosus, ischiocavernosus, superficial transverse perineal, external, anal sphincter.

- **Layer 2.** Known as the urogenital group, this group of muscles surrounds the genital and urinary muscles and is responsible for the functioning of the bladder [3]. The muscles include: urethral sphincter (sphincter urethrae), compressor urethrae, sphincter urethral vaginalis, and deep transverse perineal.

- **Layer 3.** Known as the deep pelvic floor group, these muscles which run like a hammock from the pubic bone at the front of the body to the coccyx (tailbone) at the back of the body, and to the side walls toward the hips. The muscles include: levator ani muscle (pubococcygeus or pubovisceral, pubovaginalis, puboanalis, puborectalis, iliococcygeus), coccygeus, piriformis, obturator internus, arcus tendinous of levator ani, and arcus tendinous fasciae pelvis.

Scientific Evidence for PFM Physiotherapy

Does PFM physiotherapy actually help relieve vulvodynia symptoms? Let's take a look at the evidence.

A prospective study conducted by Gentilcore-Saulnier et al., (2009) examined women suffering from provoked vestibulodynia (vulvar pain in the vestibule that lasts for at least three months) prior to having pelvic floor physical therapy. They determined that "this cohort (group) had higher tonic surface electromyography activity in their superficial PFM as well as a heightened pain response to palpation of PFM compared with a control group of women. After eight pelvic floor physical therapy sessions, the women with vestibulodynia had less PFM responsiveness to pain, less PFM tone, improved vaginal flexibility, and improved PFM capacity" [2].

A study on the impact of PFM physiotherapy for female sexual dysfunction and chronic pelvic pain was conducted by Weiss et al. (2018), who reported that, "regular in-clinic and at-home pelvic floor muscle training augments (improves) the support function of the pelvic floor, increases blood flow, and stimulates pelvic floor muscle proprioception" [2] (awareness or perception of the position and movement of the body), thus helping a woman achieve a more intense orgasm. The study's authors also stated that,"referral to a pelvic physiotherapist should occur routinely as part of the multidisciplinary approach for all women who present with any type of vulvovaginal pain" [2].

"Research indicates that pelvic physiotherapy is safe and effective and can dramatically improve symptoms related to chronic pelvic pain and long-term pelvic floor dysfunction. Pelvic physiotherapy stimulates self-empowerment of women and supports recovery of function they may have lost due to pain and dysfunction" [2].

Another study undertaken by Sadownik et al., (2018) concluded that "behavioral change stimulated by physiotherapy that enhances the patient's bodily experience is an important aspect in improving self-efficacy and decreasing the experience of overly negative cognitions" [2]. In other words, physiotherapy can help not only with pain management, but with other negative effects of pain, like depression or anxiety.

A randomized controlled trial (an experiment which tests two subject groups using two alternate treatment methods) undertaken by Goldfinger et al., (2019) "emphasized the efficacy (benefit) of PFM physiotherapy as part of the multidisciplinary approach for chronic pelvic pain and sexual dysfunction" [2]. The research team stated that to improve sexual dysfunction and chronic pelvic pain, patients need to undergo "physiotherapist-assisted stretching of all muscles related to the pelvis, abdomen, low back and upper legs, in addition to nerve gliding to facilitate movement in restricted nerves" [2]. They also reported that stability, balance, reduced neural stress, and painful intercourse are restored by strength training and stretching exercises, as well as by achieving the correct fascia tissue and pelvic floor muscle length [2].

Another randomized controlled trial carried out by Zoorob et al., (2014) analyzed women with sexual and pelvic pain. The authors "concluded that pelvic floor muscle physiotherapy improves sex life and decreases pain in an equivalent response to injections" [2].

In addition, Level I evidence and Grade A recommendation shows that "pelvic floor muscle training is effective in the treatment of female stress, urgency, or mixed urinary incontinence (UI). Pregnancy and especially vaginal births are established risk factors for development of UI, and stretch and tears of peripheral nerves, connective tissue, and pelvic floor muscles may contribute to weakness of the pelvic floor" [4].

Chronic pelvic pain and female sexual dysfunction are "prevalent and multi-factorial issues that threaten women's quality of life" [2]. There is no doubt that "as part of the multidisciplinary team, and because of its holistic and whole-body approach, PFM physiotherapy can contribute significantly to assessing and treating such women, and clinical and scientific research indicate its efficacy and safety" [2].

"Vulvar pain affects up to 20% of women at some point in their lives and the majority of these women have associated pelvic floor impairments. Because of the heterogeneity of the syndrome, successful treatment plans are multi-modal and include physical therapy" [7].

Why are Your PFM So Important?

Our PFM are important for many reasons, including the following:

- Squeezing and lifting your PFM generates sexual arousal and sensation.

- For mothers, the PFM support the baby throughout pregnancy and help during childbirth.

- Along with the core muscles of the back and abdomen, the PFM support and stabilize your spine.

- If your PFM are weak or do not function optimally over a period of time, your rectum, bladder or uterus can drop significantly and bulge (prolapse) into the vagina, causing urinary, and in some cases, faecal incontinence.

- When your small intestine or rectum is no longer supported by your PFM, it can lead to constipation [3].

It's essential for your PFM to be able to contract in order to sustain continence, and it's important for them to be able to relax during urination, bowel movements, and sexual intercourse. Holding too much muscular tension in the region can prevent these vital actions, and can cause pelvic pain, bowel and bladder urgency, and irregular frequency. If the muscles in this region are low tone (weak or hypotonic), they can contribute to organ prolapse and stress incontinence. Alternately, if your PFM are over-stressed or over-relaxed, that can also lead to problems [3].

How can you tell if your PFM are overactive (hypertonic)? If they are, you may experience some of these symptoms:

- Uncoordinated muscle contractions which cause spasm in the pelvic floor muscles

- Pain at the time of or after sexual stimulation, intercourse, or orgasm

- Inexplicable pain in the genital region, rectum, hips, pelvic area, groin or lower back

- Painful bowel movements, IBS symptoms, stomach pain, diarrhoea, straining, and constipation

- Painful urination, stopping and starting the stream of urine, burning, incomplete emptying, hesitancy, double voiding, urgency, and abnormal frequency [3]

How Does a PFMD Diagnosis Work?

"Assessing the pelvic floor without doing an internal exam is like a physiotherapist doing a knee exam through a pair of jeans. Treating any other part of the body without touching the affected body part to see which muscles are tight, or weak and how the joints move and glide, would be completely unacceptable" [5].

PFMD should only be diagnosed by a physiotherapist or doctor who specializes in this field [2]. Before starting the physical examination, the physiotherapist will help you feel at ease, tell you about the nature of the process, and set distinct boundaries.

While your physiotherapist may need to examine the painful area, they will take your pain into account and be very wary of causing you any additional pain. Before beginning an examination, your physiotherapist will ask you which areas are sore and whether touching the sore area tends to make the pain worse. They will then proceed with caution, avoiding the painful areas as much as possible and doing their best to keep you comfortable.

Diagnostic Tests for PFMD

To diagnose PFMD, your doctor or physiotherapist may perform something called an orthopedic examination, followed by a PFM exam. These tests may sound complicated, but they mainly involve the physiotherapist observing your range of motion and are usually performed without the use of any machines or x-rays. They may also involve the physiotherapist asking you questions about the nature and length of your pain.

Once the physiotherapist has carried out a full assessment of your biomechanics and alignment observing posture, and the stability of your pelvis and spine with special tests they will commence the pelvic floor muscle examination, starting by asking you to lie in the supine position (on your back), so that your abdominal wall and breathing can be assessed. The physiotherapist will examine your perineal region, taking note of your skin temperature, color, moisture level, irregularities, scars, asymmetry, hemorrhoids, skin tags etc.

This is followed by a neuromuscular assessment. This includes a skin-rolling test, hyperalgesia (Wartenberg pinwheel), pain points, and nerve entrapment. Palpation is used to examine the tone (muscular activity) of the abdominal muscles, legs, hips, and lower back. Biofeedback and/or internal palpation is employed to assess your pelvic floor's muscular tone, activity, spasm, and relaxation [6]. Some pelvic health physiotherapists will sometimes assess the patient in standing to review how the muscles of the pelvis adapt to a functional movement. Other tests your physiotherapist may perform include a neuro exam, sensation testing, and Q-tip testing.

Underlying Health Problems

As part of your diagnosis, your physiotherapist will ask for information about any underlying health issues you may have. They will also make sure you understand terms like the following: "chronic pelvic pain pathophysiology and female sexual dysfunction; involvement of pelvic floor muscles (PFM), healthy vulvovaginal and sexual behaviors, factors influencing pain intensity, relaxation techniques, sexual function, and recovery of nonpainful sexual activities" [5].

"Physiotherapist-assisted stretching of the muscles of the back, lower extremities and abdomen, in addition to nerve gliding to facilitate movement in restricted nerves, is important" [6].

Physiotherapy Treatment Methods

After diagnosis, the physiotherapist will teach you stretching, lengthening, and strengthening techniques designed to target underactive or short and stiff muscles that may be weak, to develop stability and balance. As we'll discuss later on, central sensitization and myofascial involvement may contribute to chronic pain and its related sexual dysfunction. For this reason, physiotherapists target "treatment of myofascial trigger points (MTrPs), and pain regions, especially those that have been clinically tested and enhanced by scientific studies" [6].

Treatment methods often include hands-on and visualization techniques designed to help you reconnect with your body. "These strategies are often highly valued by patients because of the careful and gradual approach, which encourages women to be active participants in the overall process" [2]. Your physiotherapist will respond to your "immediate complaints of sexual discomfort, using body work to encourage [you] to feel more in control during the procedures and sexual activities. Patients have described the body work as therapeutic and empowering" [2].

Soft Tissue Mobilization and Myofascial Release

The main physiotherapy approach to treating overactive PFM is soft tissue mobilization (STM), a common type of which is myofascial release (MFR).

Myofascial release is a physiotherapy procedure that includes a broad spectrum of treatments, including joint mobilization, stretching, deep-pressure massage, and foam rollers. It may also include other trigger-point release techniques like transversal or flat palpation, dry needling, and vibration.

When you attend a session, you'll also spend time developing techniques to increase flexibility, improve balance and stability, and lessen trigger point related tension and pain [6].

Other types of soft tissue mobilization include effleurage (a circular massage) stroke transvaginally to release tension, resolve myofascial trigger points, and lengthen PFM to their normal resting position. One exercise done in the clinic that can also be performed at home is called a "reverse Kegel." It involves bearing down gently as if trying to pass gas.

Your physiotherapist may also have you perform exercises like holding a muscle in a stretched position for a few seconds, contracting a muscle without moving, and relaxing while breathing out.

Other Strategies for Pain Management

Other management techniques involve general relaxation and respiratory exercises and working to increase your self-empowerment and self-management skills. Research conducted by Aredo et al., notes "This dual approach addresses physiological and psychological components of chronic myofascial pain, alleviates myofascial trigger point (MTrP) related pain, and gives patients coping strategies to redirect their focus during a painful episode" [2].

Other common treatment methods include Pilates and balloons for dilation of the vaginal tissue, electrical stimulation, biofeedback, and PFM pain management techniques [2].

Goldstein et al., conducted a study with the goal of restoring tissue length and PFM, thus reducing dyspareunia (pain with intercourse) and neural tension. This study referred to a vulvodynia PFM training program that included "pelvic and core mobilization and stabilization techniques; connective tissue, visceral, and neural mobilization; and internal and external myofascial trigger point release" [2].

In the study, electrical stimulation and biofeedback helped to lower the participants' tissue restrictions and sensitive points. The authors observed that "vaginal dilators are recommended to normalize muscle tone, desensitize hypersensitive areas of vulva and vagina, and restore sexual function" [2].

Pelvic Floor Physical Modalities

In addition to these methods, other practices like "electrostimulation, biofeedback, vaginal dilators or vaginal weighted cones can be used to help with isolation of pelvic floor musculature and improve contraction" [6]. Transcutaneous electrical nerve stimulation (TENS) uses a mild electrical current to deliver pain relief, through the use of electrodes placed on the skin.

Biofeedback uses a rectal or vaginal pressure sensor to deliver an audio and/or visual signal [6]. "When a pelvic floor physical therapist teaches a patient to do active pelvic floor relaxation or to breathe diaphragmatically and informs the patient of the quality of her performance, this is biofeedback" [8]. We'll discuss biofeedback in greater detail in the next chapter.

Creating and Implementing a Personalized Treatment Plan

Your physiotherapist will create a personalized treatment plan for you. This plan will likely include "relaxation and respiratory exercises, PFM training, stretching techniques, and the use of vaginal dilators, if indicated" [2]. As you continue with your treatment plan, your physiotherapist will make any necessary modifications along the way to ensure that you receive optimal treatment according to your needs.

Self-Care at Home

As with many medical conditions, self-care plays a crucial role in treating PFMD. Your physiotherapist will give you a tailor-made home exercise program, providing clear guidance as to what you need to do [2]. They may also suggest keeping a pain diary.

Learning About Persistent Pain

Your physiotherapist should provide information about how you can manage constant vulvar pain at home, and it's important to learn all you can on this subject. Not just learn it, but try to practice it. They may also discuss ways you can manage the psychological effects of pain, helping you control anxiety and negative thoughts [2].

Avoiding Strain on the Pelvic Floor Muscles

Your physiotherapist may also counsel you to make some lifestyle changes, if necessary, to avoid further weaking the PFM. There are many factors that can affect your PFM health and may lead to the muscles becoming weaker. These include:

- Weight: If you are overweight, losing some weight can help take the strain off your PFM [3].

- Constipation: Whenever the bowel is full, it exerts pressure on the bladder. If you strain or push to empty your bowel, your PFM will weaken [3].

- Smoking: In addition to its other detrimental effects, smoking can lead to coughing, which strains the pelvic muscles [3,9].

- Lifting: When lifting heavy items, especially if you do so regularly, contract your PFM to avoid straining them [3].

- Excessive lifting in the gym or for exercise. Reviewing your lifting and exercise routine with your pelvic health physiotherapist is important to reduce the impact on the pelvic floor.

- Reviewing exercises that may put pressure or irritate the pelvic floor or associated muscle e.g static bike.

How Can I Find a Pelvic Health Physiotherapist?

Physiotherapy involves "using knowledge and skills unique to a physiotherapist, and is the service only provided by, or under the direction and supervision of, a physiotherapist" [10]. In other words, you should seek out a licensed physiotherapist to help you with PFMD. Working to improve your PFM under the guidance of a physiotherapist will help ensure that the process is safe and effective.

If your physician recommends that you see a pelvic health physiotherapist, you can either search for a registered practitioner yourself (see the websites listed below) or ask your doctor for a referral.

According to the International Classification of Functions (ICF) guidelines for pelvic physiotherapy, "physiotherapists try to influence the consequences of pelvic pain and sexual dysfunction on three different levels":

- Organ: impairment/disorder level e.g. vaginal pain at penetration

- Personal: disability level e.g. inability to have intercourse

- Social: restriction of participation e.g. avoidance of sexual relationship, behavioral consequence

Do not feel embarrassed about asking for this type of guidance and treatment. Pelvic health physiotherapists have undergone a substantial degree of training and have plenty of experience in treating women with vulvodynia. They are there to help you [2].

"An estimated 16% to 25% of women with chronic pelvic pain experience dyspareunia (pain on intercourse) often leading to sexual avoidance. High pelvic floor muscle tone and sexual dysfunction are related. In women with pelvic floor dysfunction there is a positive association between pelvic floor strength and sexual activity and function" [11].

Useful Websites

In the US, information about how to find a pelvic health physiotherapist can be found on

The American Physical Therapy Association (APTA) Pelvic Health site at:

https://ptl.womenshealthapta.org/

In the UK, visit:

https://pelvicphysiotherapy.com/list-of-therapists/

https://pogp.csp.org.uk/information-patients

https://www.squeezyapp.com/directory/

Chronic pelvic pain and female sexual dysfunction are "prevalent and multi-factorial issues that threaten women's quality of life" [2]. There is no doubt that "as part of the multidisciplinary team, and because of its holistic and whole-body approach, pelvic physiotherapy can contribute significantly to assessing and treating such women, and clinical and scientific research indicate its efficacy and safety" [2]. Physiotherapy of the kind described in this chapter can go a long way toward relieving vulvar pain and improving your quality of life.

Chapter 11

Biofeedback for Vulvodynia

"The biofeedback approach is based on the idea that women with vulvodynia and vulvar vestibulitis syndrome have unstable muscles in the walls of the pelvis. This may explain the shooting and stabbing pains often described by women with vulvodynia, as well as pain that results from touch and stimulation" [1].

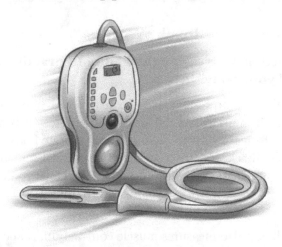

One tool your pelvic physiotherapist may use to help you find relief is a biofeedback machine. Electromyography (EMG) biofeedback, usually just referred to as biofeedback, can be helpful for treating women's pelvic pain and sexual dysfunction issues [2].

Why is biofeedback used to treat vulvodynia? According to one theory, muscle over-activity can cause your muscles to be continually contracted. Over time, this brings tight pelvic floor muscles, generating nerve compression and irritation, and, ultimately, vulvar pain [1]. Biofeedback training can help you connect with your pelvic floor muscles (PFM) and learn how to relax them. In fact, it may be one of the most promising supplementary physical therapies in this area.

Once you have control of your PFM and can easily contract and release them, you can move on to strengthen the weakened muscles [1].

"Biofeedback-based or biofeedback-augmented interventions have the potential to serve as treatments for sexual dysfunction concerns, especially among women, for whom current psycho-social treatments are lacking" [2].

Some biofeedback software is specifically engineered for vulvodynia sufferers. Instead of standard biofeedback units, which require placing electrodes on the skin, these vulvodynia units use special sensors that are gently placed into the vagina [1].

How Does Biofeedback Work?

"Biofeedback gives you the ability to practice new ways to control your body" [3].

Biofeedback is a system used to teach you how to relax and exercise certain muscles. As the Mayo Clinic notes "it is a technique you can use to learn how to control some of your body's functions. During biofeedback, you are connected to electrical sensors that help you receive information about your body. This helps you make subtle changes in your body, such as relaxing certain muscles to reduce pain" [3].

Biofeedback also measures muscle contraction. A special vaginal sensor linked to an electromyograph (EMG) monitors the electrical activity generating the muscular contraction [3]. An EMG is a standard diagnostic tool that assesses the condition of muscles and the nerve cells (motor neurons) that regulate them. Motor neurons are responsible for transmitting the electrical signals which make our muscles relax and contract [3].

Using Computer Graphics and Prompts

Biofeedback uses computer graphics and prompts to empower you to manage your stress levels by relaxing your muscles, pacing your breathing, and thinking positively about your situation. Research indicates that these methods "might be effective in improving responses during stressful periods; and inducing feelings of calm and well-being" [3].

What Can I Expect During a Biofeedback Session?

Most biofeedback sessions last 30 to 60 minutes. At the start of the session, your therapist will attach small electrical sensors, like ECG stickers, onto a bony area, normally your knee or hip. This gives the machine a base line of no muscle contraction.

You will then insert a small sensor probe into your vagina. Next, your therapist will ask you to do a set of contractions and relaxations, and show you a screen where you can see what your pelvic floor is doing [3].

The electrical sensors and sensor probe send data cues back to the machine, cues like a flashing light, bleeping sound, or other changes on the monitor. This feedback prompts you to change your behavior, thought processes, and emotions, ultimately empowering you to control or adjust the way your body responds to pain and muscle spasm [3].

The therapist will then teach you how to "make deliberate physical changes in your body, such as relaxing specific muscles, to reduce your pain" [3]. Once you're comfortable with these techniques, you can continue practicing in the comfort of your own home [3].

The number and length of biofeedback sessions you may need depend on your unique situation, as well as how long it takes you to master your physical responses.

Why Biofeedback?

Many people like biofeedback for the following reasons:

- It is not invasive.
- It may reduce the need for medications.
- It may enhance the benefits of medications.

- It empowers people to take more control over their health [3].

The Limitations of Biofeedback

Of course, biofeedback has its limits. "Even if a pelvic floor physical therapist uses EMG to relax the pelvic floor muscles, this is often not enough to fully lengthen the muscle fibers. Manual input into the muscle fibers, that is, pressure and stretch, helps to bring proper blood flow and oxygen to overactive pelvic floor muscles" [6].

Biofeedback alone cannot bring full relief and healing. When a woman's pelvic floor muscles are extremely tight and short "the EMG biofeedback cannot read the contraction, with the biofeedback screen displaying a flat line. This leaves the provider and patient nothing to work with" [6].

Can Biofeedback Work as a Stand-Alone Therapy?

While biofeedback can be extremely helpful, it's most effective when combined with other treatment methods, such as pelvic floor exercises and soft tissue mobilization.

"It is important to emphasize that biofeedback is not at its most effective when used as a treatment alone but should be integrated with other therapeutic interventions. It acts as an enhancer of the therapy, enabling the patient and therapist to make more effective and rapid progress towards the rehabilitation goal" [7].

According to one study "Biofeedback is well-accepted as a primary or adjunct treatment for specific sexual concerns in women. However, biofeedback would likely be best utilized as part of a multidimensional treatment model, including psychological, pharmacological, and surgical steps. Future research may better determine the precise role of biofeedback in multi-component treatment protocols" [2].

Your physiotherapist can help you decide whether biofeedback will work for your situation.

Where Can I Get Biofeedback Therapy?

You can find registered, licensed biofeedback therapists at various hospitals, medical centers, and physiotherapy clinics. If you're not sure where to start, try doing a Google search for biofeedback therapists in your area. Many are licensed in another field of health care, such as physiotherapy, nursing, or psychology [3].

A Look at the Broader Meaning of Biofeedback

If you're confused about the meaning of biofeedback, you're not alone. The term "biofeedback" can carry multiple meanings, and in addition to the computer-based treatment program, is used to refer to the following:

1. Whenever a medic gives feedback on your active PFM contraction.

2. When a pelvic floor physical therapist uses a finger to determine whether you are relaxing or tensing, and then informs you.

3. When a pelvic floor physical therapist teaches you to breathe diaphragmatically and informs you about the quality of the performance.

4. When a pelvic floor therapist asks you to do an active pelvic floor relaxation, and then gives you feedback on how to improve this activity [6].

Pelvic physiotherapists frequently use biofeedback to help women suffering from pelvic pain and female sexual dysfunction [8]. As discussed, it is not used as a stand-alone treatment, but as an addition to other, more general treatment methods.

Chapter 12

Desensitization using Dilators and Vibrators for Vulvodynia

"**Because pelvic floor muscle disorders contribute significantly to chronic pelvic pain and sexual dysfunction, there is rationale for physiotherapy. However, physiotherapy is a widely underused and untapped resource, which has its place in the multidisciplinary approach to these health problems**" [1].

Muscle desensitization is another technique your physiotherapist may recommend. This can be carried out using vaginal dilators (also known as vaginal trainers), or vibrators, as we'll discuss in this chapter.

With muscle desensitization treatment, it's crucial to follow the guidance you are given by your pelvic physiotherapist. If you are experiencing painful sex, then desensitizing your vagina muscles is vital for managing your condition [2].

Desensitizing the Vaginal Region

One technique for gently desensitizing the region and stretching out contracted vaginal tissue is to progressively introduce larger items into your vagina. You might start by using your finger, then your partner's finger, then a very small vaginal trainer. If you find that just using your finger is painful, use a little olive oil or lubricant to make things easier. Carry out this process as many times as your therapist recommends per week [2].

It's easy to give up and assume that stretching out your vaginal tissue is impossible. But even if you manage to get part of your finger inserted, you will have made a good start. Think of it as a tiny first step on the way to getting your vagina back to optimum condition. Remember that the results you are working toward will take time.

Your physiotherapist may recommend this exercise along with one or more medical treatments. They may also suggest that you incorporate pelvic floor exercises with a dilator and/or vibrator.

"The protective guarding response that can occur in women with vulvar pain needs to be unlearned, so that the body begins to remember that inserting something into the vagina does not need to be painful" [2].

Vaginal Dilators

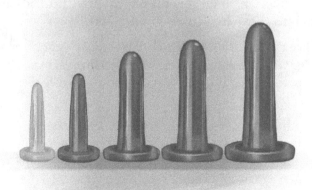

Also known as vaginal trainers, vaginal dilators are smooth-textured silicone or plastic cylinders, designed to be inserted into the vagina one at a time to help penetration. They are engineered to help you gently stretch and desensitize the region and relax the muscles around the vagina's entrance. Dilators can also help you feel less anxious about being touched in that region [4].

Vaginal dilators are available in a set of different sizes. This way, you can start with a small one and slowly work your way up to the larger ones, as and when you feel comfortable [4].

How Do I Use Dilators?

Ideally, you want to use dilators under the advice of your pelvic health physiotherapist. This ensures that you have a personalized program to follow, and it may also help to boost your motivation [2].

Start with the smallest dilator. Your therapist may recommend a lubricant that you can lightly coat the dilator with before use. Be sure to get a recommendation before applying the lubricant, as some lubricants contain chemicals that could irritate your condition and cause your tissues to react [2].

Very gently, insert the tip of the smallest dilator into your vagina. Supporting the dilator with your hand, leave it in place for 5 to 10 minutes. Then, when you're ready, try repeating this process but inserting half of the dilator, then the whole dilator. After you're comfortable with inserting the whole dilator, you can move on to the next size, repeating the same technique.

Your physiotherapist will instruct you as to how many times per week or day you should conduct this exercise. Before moving on through the different sizes, rate your pain level and self-confidence with each size. You can do this by filling out a pain diary, which you can then show to your physiotherapist, who will be able to rate your progression. The therapist may introduce breathing techniques and stretches to assist with dilator training either in the session or for patient personal practice.

How Long Should the Dilator Stay Inserted?

When it comes to how long you should keep the dilator in your vagina, this is generally "the same on each occasion, around 10 minutes. Some women feel more conscious of the pelvic floor muscles if they contract and then relax them around the dilator" [2], so you may wish to try this.

Hygiene

It's essential to keep the dilators clean. After each use, clean the dilator according to the manufacturers' instructions. Often, this simply involves applying warm, soapy water and then drying it off. No special cleansers are usually required.

Dilators versus Vibrators

"Medical dilators can help to stretch the tight tissues of the vagina whilst a vibrator can promote blood flow to the healing tissues and feel pleasurable too, especially on the clitoris" [4].

In the past, many women chose to use a standard vibrator, or even self-massage their vulvar region, instead of using a clinical, hard plastic dilator. But these days, dilators are also available in soft silicone; and several offer a vibration option [4].

Many women don't want to use vibrators because they regard them as sexual toys, as opposed to medical aids. Others find a vibrator less sexual. After months or years of medical interventions and treatment, some women want to feel sexual again [4]. There is a happy medium, since both vibrators and dilators "can be used in conjunction with each other, as they offer different experiences for many women" [4].

The best approach is to keep an open mind. Be willing to try both options, but follow your physiotherapist's guidance regarding which method is best for you.

Chapter 13

Pelvic Floor Training Chairs for Vulvodynia

Pelvic Floor Training Chairs use magnetic field therapy to tone and improve your pelvic musculature, helping to treat and improve weak or dysfunctional pelvic muscles. In this chapter, we'll discuss three types of Pelvic Floor Training Chairs:

- The Pelvic Floor Training Chair for Magnetic Field Therapy (MFT)
- The Pelvic Floor Chair for Biofeedback
- The BTL Emsella Chair

The Pelvic Floor Training Chair for Magnetic Field Therapy (MFT)

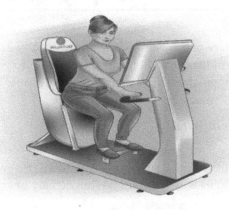

This resembles a comfortable reclining chair. Patients simply sit (fully clothed) on the pelvic chair for 15 minutes. A minimum of four 15-minute sessions are recommended, depending on the program, and treatment time can vary between one to six months.

Each session is programmed to provide you with optimal treatment for your condition. During the session, a physiotherapist or specialist nurse makes any necessary adjustments. After each session, you remain seated and rest in the therapy chair for five minutes [1].

How Does it Work?

"Passive training with RPMS (repetitive peripheral muscle stimulation) can precede active training for patients who cannot willingly contract their pelvic floor because it is not strong enough" [1].

During Pelvic Floor Training for MFT, the training system relays sensory data to your brain, generating long-term neurological changes. This increases "personal awareness of, and the ability to control, and indirectly coordinate individual muscle functions" [1].

Repetitive peripheral muscle stimulation (RPMS) excites the muscles of the pelvic floor on a neuromuscular level. Acting as a micro-massage, RPMS circulates throughout the lower lumbar region (vertebrae in the lower back) and trunk, stimulating the muscles. If you have scarring or slight fascial adhesions, RPMS could help resolve these [1].

Because RPMS therapy activates the entire circulatory system, it's ideal for anyone who wants to strengthen their pelvic floor and experience neuromuscular training in an easy, effective way [1].

Seat Action

The seat surface of this chair incorporates stimulation technology, generating vertical magnetic field impulses of up to 2 teslas. Due to this action, this type of training provides significantly greater results than you could ever gain by just training alone [1].

Getting Technical

To get technical for a moment, the stimulation system, along with the affiliated electronics, provide "repetitive magnetic impulses lasting 200 to 500 µs with a magnetic flux density of approx. 0.5 tesla and the maximum field strength at the coil of up to 2 teslas. The electric induction elicits electrical potential shifts in the overlying tissue that are so pronounced as to bring about depolarisation of the peripheral nerves. The resulting action potential of the depolarised nerves leads to contractions of the connected muscles. Each impulse generates an individual contraction or a brief muscle spasm" [1].

What Does the Science Say?

Scientific studies show that the Pelvic Floor Training Chair for MFT is "more effective than standard individual training" [1].

Winfried Mayr, professor for biomedical engineering and rehabilitation technology at the Medical University of Vienna, states "Magnetic field stimulation is a proven alternative to traditional electro-therapy. Electro-therapy always involves intervention in the most intimate parts of our bodies and must be performed using invasive electrodes. In contrast, Pelvic Floor Training Chair ensures a more pleasant experience for the patient and the attending physician or therapist and takes a lot less time" [1].

Research in the American *Journal of Urology* (2017) says that "The effectiveness of the magnetic field stimulation of muscles, especially of the pelvic floor, was demonstrated decades ago and has been investigated in major and smaller studies worldwide" [2].

All the evidence, then, points to the Pelvic Floor Training Chair for MFT being effective.

The Pelvic Floor Chair for Biofeedback

The Pelvic Floor Chair for Biofeedback resembles an indoor sports bike without pedals. Sessions last 10 minutes, and you're given a personalised plan as to how many sessions you need. This machine is perfect for anyone who cannot participate in magnetic field training, for example, because they are pregnant or have metal in their body [1].

The Pelvic Floor Chair for Biofeedback Training is designed to support your independent training. As discussed in the previous chapter, biofeedback is a technique that uses auditory or visual feedback to help you gain control of your bodily functions. Your therapist works to retrain your pelvic floor muscles, so that your muscles relax and strengthen according to your individual needs [1].

"The monitor visualises the patient's independent training/recruitment of their pelvic floor. Their body awareness is improved and enhanced in a playful setting" [1].

The pelvic floor lifts and tenses while you train, and this tension is held for a certain period before the muscles relax. The exercise cycles are repeated a few times [1].

How Does it Work?

You can undergo training in a relaxed, seated position with an adjustable backrest. An integrated sensor detects the activity of your pelvic floor muscles. At each training, the sensor provides on-screen visualisation of your muscle movements via a monitor situated in front of you. The biofeedback raises your self-awareness of your pelvic floor, as well as the strength of the training [1]. Naturally, being able to see this process in action can be very encouraging.

What Does the Science Say?

Fresenius-Hochschule of Germany evaluated the Pelvic Floor Chair's functionality using EMG measurement. This incorporated the musculature of the pelvic floor, along with the activity of three other muscle groups (the long adductor, the gluteus maximus, and the internal obliques).

"For all subjects, the findings demonstrate clear evidence for training of the pelvic floor using the Bio-Feedback-Trainer. It is therefore, a very suitable device to train the pelvic floor musculature. The study proved that the biofeedback function enables tracking of the pelvic floor activity without intimate contact" [1]. Clearly, the idea of effective treatment without intimate contact is something which will be a relief to many people, especially vulvodynia sufferers.

Note: The Pelvic Floor Chair for Biofeedback Training is also known as the Pelvic Floor Bike-Like Chair for Biofeedback Training and the Pelvic Floor Training Chair Biofeedback.

The BTL Emsella Chair

"Electromagnetic stimulation of the sacral nerve roots and pelvic floor continues to evolve as a non-invasive treatment alternative for pelvic floor dysfunction" [3].

The Emsella chair is designed to stimulate the pelvic floor's total musculature. This is in sharp contrast to what can be achieved by doing Kegel exercising, which only works on a particular muscular subset.

The great news is that spending just half an hour in the Emsella chair is the equivalent of doing 11,000 pelvic floor exercises. This chair enables some women to feel their pelvic floor muscles tensing and relaxing [3].

While you may see positive results after only two or three half-hour treatments; in most cases, the best outcome is achieved by a course of six sessions over a three-week span. In rare cases, more sessions are needed, but most of the time, a maintenance session, repeated at intervals from between three months to one year, is sufficient [3].

Chapter 14

Can a Nerve Block Relieve Vulvodynia?

"Women who have long-standing pain that doesn't respond to other treatments might benefit from local nerve block injections" [1].

Vulvodynia is a form of neuropathic, or nerve, pain. As such, nerve block treatment is one possible solution for vulvodynia. Some of these treatments focus on the pudendal nerve, which we'll discuss below, but other types of nerve treatment can also be successful.

"Women suffering from vulvodynia may experience sharp, burning, or electric shock-like pain that can occur around the vulva, labia or entrance to the vagina. Researchers agree that nerve dysfunction is common, and the pudendal nerve is the main nerve that supplies this area, so more advanced treatment for nerve pain is targeted here" [2].

The Pudendal Nerve

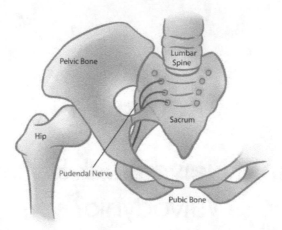

The pudendal nerve is located at the back of the pelvis and extends to near your vagina. At this point, it branches into other nerves. The pudendal nerve communicates with the perineum, anus, urethra, and external genitals. It controls some of the muscles in your bladder and around your anus, in other words, the muscles that allow you to use the bathroom [3]. If you're experiencing vulvar pain, the issue could be connected to your pudendal nerve, and targeting this nerve may help to relieve your pain.

What is a Pudendal Nerve Block?

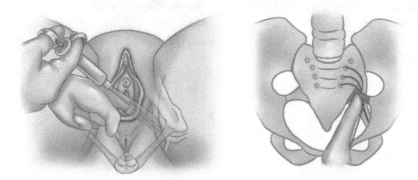

There are two types of pudendal nerve blocks. Diagnostic pudendal nerve blocks help physicians diagnose nerve dysfunction, while the purpose of therapeutic pudendal nerve blocks is to provide pain relief.

In a diagnostic pudendal nerve block, a local anesthetic is administered to the pudendal nerve. Since the pudendal nerve carries pain signals from the vulva and perineum (the area between the anus and vulva) to the spine, this procedure can help the physician find out if your vulvodynia is connected to your pudendal nerve. If it is, then steroids and radiofrequency treatment may help relieve your pain.

A therapeutic pudendal nerve block is similar, but in this procedure, the local anesthetic is combined with a corticosteroid, for example methylprednisolone, triamcinolone or dexamethasone. Corticosteroids reduces nerve irritation and blocks certain nerves. It takes about 10 to 14 days to work, but can provide pain relief for several months [2].

"After 10-14 days, there is often a very significant reduction in pain, with up to 60-65% of patients feeling better" [2].

At the London Pain Clinic, patients are given local anesthetic to make the procedure pain-free, with the option of light sedation to ensure it is as relaxing and well tolerated as possible. "The area is cleaned with a sterile solution. Using image guidance, the physician inserts a needle through the skin and deeper tissues. The patient is then monitored for a minimum of 30 minutes following the procedure, after which, they are free to return home" [2].

In general, nerve blocks are very safe procedures. Negative effects like local bleeding, bruising, infection, and discomfort are possible but uncommon. Sexual, bowel, and bladder dysfunction do not occur, and nerve damage is very rare. If nerve damage does occur, it's usually temporary and most patients recover fully within weeks.

Other Types of Nerve Block for Patients Suffering from Vulvodynia

Pudendal Nerve Pulsed Radiofrequency (PRF)

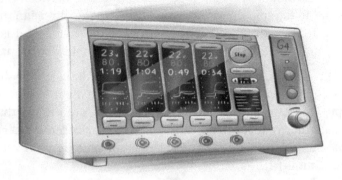

If a pudendal nerve block is successful, but longer lasting pain relief is required, your doctor may recommend pudendal nerve pulsed radiofrequency treatment, or PRF. This procedure is similar to the pudendal nerve block, but instead of injecting medications through a needle, the physician will treat the pudendal nerve with pulsed radiofrequency, a non-destructive electrical treatment for nerves. This has been shown to improve nerve function and relieve pain for anywhere from 6 to 12 months or more [4].

As with pudendal nerve block treatment, this procedure is very safe and negative effects are rare, though local bleeding, bruising, infection, and discomfort can occur. Nerve damage from the procedure is very rare and usually temporary.

Sacral Nerve Root Block

If your pain is more widespread, or if a pudendal nerve block has only provided partial relief, you may want to try a sacral nerve root block. As with a pudendal nerve block, there are two types: diagnostic and therapeutic.

A diagnostic sacral nerve root block is much like a pudendal nerve block, but it targets the sacral nerve root. Using an x-ray, the physician inserts the needle into the skin of the buttock over the sacrum and administers a local anesthetic. They can then determine if your vulvodynia is connected to the sacral nerve roots, and if so, they can plan further treatments with corticosteroids or pulsed radiofrequency treatment.

A therapeutic nerve block administers a corticosteroid preparation to the sacral nerve roots. Like a therapeutic pudendal nerve block, it usually takes 10 to 14 days to work, then relieves pain for several months [2].

Benefits and side effects are the same as for a pudendal nerve block, as described above.

Sacral Nerve Root Pulsed Radiofrequency (PRF)

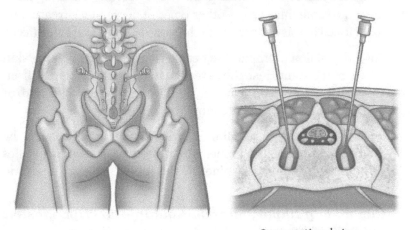

Posterior view   Cross sectional view

A sacral nerve root pulsed radiofrequency, or PRF, is basically the same as a pudendal nerve PRF, but targeting the sacral nerve root instead of the pudendal nerve. It's used when a sacral nerve root block is successful, but longer lasting pain relief is required. Your physician will place probes around the sacral nerve roots and use pulsed radiofrequency to provide pain relief for around 6 to 12 months or more.

PRF won't change the feeling of the skin and will not affect the function of your bladder or bowels.

Ganglion of Impar, Superior and Inferior Hypogastric Blocks

A ganglion is a collection of nerves. The ganglions listed above control the functions of the pelvis, bladder, upper vagina, uterus, ovaries, and rectum; but they can also transmit pain from these areas. That means your vulvodynia may be connected to these ganglions, especially if you're also experiencing changes in your bladder or bowel function. If this is the case, an injection to these ganglions may relieve your pain.

Diagnostic and therapeutic blocks that target these ganglions can help diagnose and relieve vulvar pain. They're performed using an x-ray along the same lines as the other types of nerve block treatments we've discussed in this chapter, with the same benefits and side effects.

For the ganglion of impar, the needle is inserted through the skin at the base of the spine, just above the tailbone. You may benefit from this treatment if your pain is mostly at the back of the pelvis and/or anus. Relief can last for several months.

Since the hypogastric ganglion is located higher up, just below the waist on both sides of the spine, this procedure uses two needles placed on either side of the spine. Again, relief can last for several months.

Ganglion of Impar, Superior and Inferior Hypogastric Pulsed Radiofrequency (PRF)

If a ganglion block is successful but a longer duration of pain relief is required, you may benefit from pulsed radiofrequency (PRF) treatment. Like the other types of PRFs discussed above, this procedure can offer relief for around 6 to 12 months. Benefits and side effects are the same as for other PRF treatments.

Dynamic Quadripolar Radio Frequency (DQRF)

This cutting-edge technology, which is referred to as DQRF, was developed by a biotech company in Italy. It was then specifically adapted for the purpose of treating vulvodynia sufferers, and later incorporated into a low-energy, DQRF-based EVA (Enhancement Vaginal Anatomy) device. In addition to improving the pain, DQRF is also geared to anatomically re-model the tissues in a woman's vulva, and thus indirectly reconstruct a woman's vaginal and vestibular ecosystem [5].

This device enables the DQRF generator's reduced energy flow to interact with deep tissue in the vestibule and vagina. Using the electronically driven temperature and movement sensors on the device, a practitioner can easily control the vestibular temperature of the deep tissue [5].

Research

Previous research had been done on DQRF technology's vulvar remodeling capabilities, and researchers wondered if these previous findings could help with managing localized provoked vulvodynia (LPV). To learn more, they conducted a study on a group of 30 childbearing-age women who suffered from recurrent vulvovaginal candidiasis (RVVC, also known as yeast infection) and/or recurrent aerobic vaginitis (RAV, a type of vaginal infection) [5].

Researchers wanted to determine whether or not "remodeling of vestibular and vaginal tissues, beyond its established aesthetic value in women with variable degrees of vulvovaginal hypotrophy, could also help to restore a more physiological vestibular and vaginal ecology and influence the Lactobacillus microflora to its normal role" [5].

In other words, researchers were trying to discover whether or not they could use DQRF to reconstruct vestibular and vaginal tissues and ultimately reduce vulvar pain.

Method

The women in the study received treatment in line with the EVA™/DQRF vulvovaginal protocol. The highest emitting frequency was 55 W. When used in an optimal mode, the four electrodes sent out "energy with high precision in the sub-epithelial layers of the vulva and allowed fine tuning of the vulvar thermal effect, in terms both of tissue volumes and depth" [5].

Results

The researchers discovered that the benefits of this method were "at least comparable to those of pelvic floor rehabilitation, and they could be even greater" [5]. This study supports the idea that "DQRF-induced tissue remodeling in certain vestibular areas may help to restore the normal Lactobacillus-dominated ecology of these areas and normalize patients' responsiveness to their perception of pain in the vestibule" [5].

The DQRF method helped to reduce participants' pain by restoring a healthy tissue structure to the vestibule and vagina. In light of that, DQRF technology could be "a promising new strategy to control provoked vulvodynia and the severe impact on female self-esteem that is all too often associated with this poorly recognized disorder" [5].

While more research is needed to identify just to what degree radiofrequency can help treat vulvodynia, it is emerging as a new possibility. Ask your clinician or physiotherapist for more information if you are interested.

Chapter 15

How Botulinum Toxin (Botox®/Dysport®) Can Help Vulvodynia

"Injection of botulinum toxin A brought a marked improvement in patients with intractable pain, which was not controlled with various conventional management programs" [1].

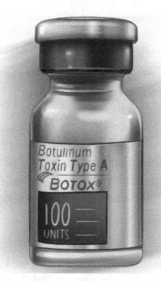

For women whose vulvodynia is due, at least in part, to muscle spasm, Botox may help relieve pain.

According to the International Journal of Obstetrics and Gynecology, Botox (specifically botulinum toxin A), can be administered without significant side effects, and "has been most extensively investigated as a possible injectable treatment for vulvodynia. In addition to a reduction in superimposed pelvic floor muscle spasm, it may also possess efficacy for vulvodynia because of its ability to inhibit substance P release, a neurotransmitter associated with inflammation and pain" [2].

How Does It Work?

Botox for vulvar pain is administered into the pelvic muscles and to localized areas of the vulva itself. For example, Botox injected into the levator ani muscles of the pelvic floor can help relieve pelvic floor muscle spasm. In addition to breaking the cycle of spasm and pain, Botox can help relax the pelvic floor muscles (PFM) to make PFM exercises easier. Other sites of injection include the bulbospongiosus muscles surrounding the vaginal opening, and just under the mucosa of the vulval vestibule.

If you suffer from provoked vestibulodynia, or provoked pain around the opening of the vagina, but do not have muscle spasm, Botox injected into these muscles may not be as effective.

Based on a number of studies, the average dose of Botox in each injection varies from 10 IU (international units) to 50 IU, and the total amount used per treatment varies from 20 IU to 100 IU or more. Sometimes the site of injection is predetermined, whereas at other times, practitioners use the distribution of pain and tenderness to guide placement of the injections. After the procedure, some women need a routine top up every two weeks, four weeks, three months, or six months. In other cases, no routine top up is needed.

What Does the Research Say?

Let's review the studies on using Botox for vulvar pain. Please note that the studies in this chapter concentrate on treatment of provoked vestibulodynia, rather than the other pain syndromes sometimes treated with Botox.

One study used a randomized, controlled trial to determine just how effective a vulvar Botox injection is. In a group of 64 women, they injected some with 10 IU of Botox, and the rest with 10 IU of saline (salt water). Guided by electromyelograph (EMG), practitioners identified the muscle fibres most in spasm within the bulbospongiosus muscle (a muscle in the pelvic floor) and injected the substance there. In this case, the saline acted as a placebo, or a harmless substance with no effect, simply used as a data point to compare with the Botox.

Both groups of women reported a significant improvement in pain. According to the visual analogue pain score (VAS), their pain levels dropped from 7.53 to 5.13 in six months. There was no significant difference between the women who received Botox and those who received saline, but this may be because the dose of Botox was small, and/or the bulbospongiosus muscle may not be the most effective site for the injection [3].

In a second randomized, controlled trial, practitioners again measured Botox against a placebo. 33 women in three groups received either 25 IU or 50 IU of Botox or placebo in each of two injection sites (located at five and seven o'clock in the submucosa of the vestibule). These sites were not the pain points, but the points at which the pudendal nerve enters the vulva.

All three groups of women showed a small improvement in pain, but there was no significant difference between the groups. The fact that there was a single predetermined injection site for all participants may have something to do with this [4].

Other studies have reported better results. In one, a series of 20 women received Botox injections into the bulbospongiosus muscle under EMG guidance, as in the first trial discussed above. The women reported that their pain scores changed from 8.37 to 2.57 in three months, and to 3.90 in six months. The treatment also improved their quality of life and sexual function, and no one reported any side effects [5]. A follow-up study reported similar results after two years [6].

Studies that focus on submucosal injections in the vulvar vestibule have similarly good results. In one of these, 11 women received up to five injections of 20 IU each. Four weeks later, five of the women received a second series of injections. Eight of the 11 women were satisfied with the results, with average pain scores dropping from 8.1 to 2.5 [7].

In a similar study that involved submucosal injections, women received top up injections, with double strength if necessary, after two weeks. Following treatment, pain scores dropped from between 8 and 10 to between 0 and 2. "In all seven patients, pain decreased or disappeared after botulinum toxin A injections... The patients reported that, after the treatment, they experienced subjective improvement in their sexual life, having no significant pain or discomfort during or after intercourse" [1].

Based on these various controlled and uncontrolled trials, especially the set of uncontrolled trials, we can conclude that Botox provides positive, encouraging results for some vulvodynia sufferers.

For provoked vestibulodynia, multiple submucosal injections totalling 100 IU units or more seem to bring the best results; and top up injections two to four weeks later appear to improve the outcome.

"Botulinum toxin therapy would be useful and safe in managing vulvodynia of muscular or neuro-inflammatory origins" [1].

Can Botox Work for You?

"Botulinum toxin A appears to be a promising option for managing sexual pain disorder" [2]. More and more data reveals that botulinum toxin A, or Botox, can decrease pain by successfully blocking the sensation of a painful stimulus through sensory nerves (this is called the superior antinociceptive effect). This effect can be used to treat long-term pain when the cause is unknown, as with vulvodynia [2].

Various studies have shown that Botox injections are effective for a good percentage of women, so if you are a suitable candidate, this form of treatment may be worth considering. Ask your doctor or physiotherapist if you want to learn more.

Chapter 16

Sacral Neuromodulation for Vulvodynia

What is Neuromodulation?

Neuromodulation is a technologically advanced method for treating disease; it uses medical devices and electric impulses to influence the activity of your nervous system. In this method, a practitioner may surgically implant a device and an insulated lead wire, the latter of which is placed along the sacral nerve roots, normally at the level of the S3 root. Via this wire, the device sends out electric impulses capable of modifying your nerve cell activity [1].

Neuromodulation is short for sacral neuromodulation (SNM) and is also known as sacral nerve stimulation (SNS).

"Although the exact mechanism of action is unknown, sacral neuromodulation may be a viable option for the management of chronic pain syndromes of the vulva and vagina" [2].

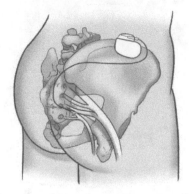

Sacral neuromodulation was first introduced into the medical profession in the nineties, and since then "has proven to be a useful treatment of chronic dysfunction of the urinary, bowel and pelvic floor" [1]. Because the sacral nerves controls your pelvic floor, bowel, and bladder, together with the corresponding muscles, modifying these nerves can help manage conditions that affect those areas [1].

The Procedure

"Patients undergo a neuromodulation trial. Those who experience reduced pain with stimulation (often defined as at least 50% reduction in pain), are then allowed to progress on to implantation of a permanent implantable pulse generator" [2].

Stage 1

In stage 1, the clinician inserts the tip of a permanent electrode into your lower back and positions it near your sacral nerve root. They join the end of this electrode to a temporary lead cable, which is tunnelled through your back (under the skin), and later removed if the test phase is successful. After implanting the electrode, the clinician connects the cable to a generator [1]. Then, the test phase or trial period begins.

The Test Phase or Trial Period

"The trial period is important, as it helps prevent placement of an expensive permanent device with its associated side effects, into a patient who may subsequently not respond to the therapy" [2].

During this period of between two to eight weeks, the clinician will assess whether you could benefit from having a sacral neuromodulation device permanently implanted.

You'll also have the chance to test out having an implant and see whether or not it impacts your day-to-day work routine and lifestyle. If you and your clinician decide that this is a good option for you, then you will move on to the second stage of the procedure, which involves implanting the permanent indwelling generator [1].

Stage 2

In stage 2, your clinician inserts the permanent generator, which is attached to the previously implanted electrode. "This (generator) is sited in a subcutaneous pocket (under the skin) in the lower quadrant of the abdomen or upper buttock and provides electrical stimulation" [2].

During this procedure, the temporary cable inserted in stage 1 is removed. As soon as the definitive generator is turned on, you may experience a similar feeling to the one you had during stage 1 [1]. Both stage 1 and stage 2 are usually performed under general or local anaesthesia.

Handheld Programmer and Medical Device Card

After successful implantation, your clinician will give you a handheld programmer and device card. It's important to carry this card with you so healthcare professionals know you have an implant [1].

What About Follow-Up Care?

Your clinician will advise you on this during the consultation part of the procedure [1].

Are There Any Potential Side Effects?

Negative side effects are possible. They include infection, pain, bleeding, and bruising in the wound area. Rarely, placing the electrodes can irritate nerves that go down to the legs, causing pain that radiates down the legs.

The hardware can also bring potential side effects. For example, there is a chance that the lead cable could break, hence the need for the surgeon to handle it carefully. If the lead is pulled, this could displace the permanent electrode, causing loss of sensation or pain. If this happens, your clinician should surgically reposition the electrode (as in stage 1) [1].

Change in Sensation

If, after time, the normal sensation disappears or changes, you may need the settings on your device adjusted. Before adjusting the settings, your clinician will check the position of the electrode, possibly using an X-ray [1].

Post-Surgery Limitations

To avoid moving the electrode, steer clear of high-intensity sports and strenuous work, including stretching and lifting weights, for a minimum of six months after surgery. Avoid doing any heavy lifting during the first three months post-surgery, particularly when that lifting involves twisting or bending [1].

Your doctor will advise you further regarding the length of the recovery period. Once this period ends, "you can do most forms of exercise, such as swimming, running, aerobics, etc. Horseback riding, skiing, and contact sports are associated with more lead or electrode breakage" [1] and are therefore not recommended.

What Happens If I Become Pregnant?

Currently, the impact of sacral neuromodulation on pregnancy is not known. If you are hoping to have a baby, or if you find out that you are pregnant, talk to your clinician. They may recommend switching off your modulator [1].

How Will Appliances Affect Me?

Occasionally, standard appliances like audio speakers and refrigerators can hinder your implant. If this happens, the implant may need to be restarted. Bear in mind that "even if the device is turned off, nearby strong electrical gadgets can still affect the lead, which could result in a sudden and brief shock or jolt" [1].

Can Neuromodulation Help Me?

Let's look at an example of how neuromodulation may help relieve vulvodynia. A 42-year-old woman suffering from chronic vulvar vestibular syndrome had had little success with other therapies. After a discussion with her medical consultant, she was offered sacral neuromodulation.

"She underwent a standard two-phase surgical implantation with good result at two years post-implantation" [3]. In the end "sacral neuromodulation was shown to be a valid treatment option for this patient and resulted in excellent patient satisfaction at two-year follow-up" [3].

Stories like this suggest that neuromodulation can help vulvodynia sufferers, but as with some of the other treatments discussed in this book, more research is needed.

Currently, most studies on neuromodulation relate to other conditions, which is not helpful for those suffering from vulvodynia, nor for the doctors advising them. Further, as most doctors in clinical practice do not have primary training in neuromodulation "it may be difficult for them to decide when neuromodulation is appropriate..." [2].

To determine the benefits of neuromodulation and learn which vulvodynia sufferers are likely to get the best outcomes "larger prospective randomized studies with carefully selected patient groups are required" [2]. Indeed "the use of neuromodulation for various chronic pelvic pain syndromes is still in its experimental phase, and a matter of considerable debate" [2].

If you are interested in this treatment method, talk to your doctor or clinician. They may be able to recommend a neuromodulation consultant who can give you further information.

Chapter 17

Foods and Supplements for Vulvodynia

You've probably heard the saying "you are what you eat," and nutrition can play a significant role in your health, so it's no surprise that diet may affect your vulvodynia symptoms. Some studies suggest that cutting out foods like gluten and dairy can help reduce vulval pain, as can adding supplements like probiotics.

Then again, it's important to realize that research in this area is still limited, and everyone has different food sensitivities. In other words, what works for one person may or may not work for you. Still, the nutritional approach is definitely worth exploring.

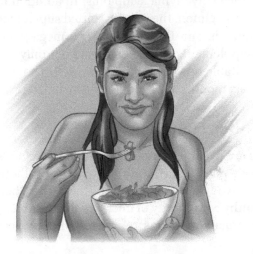

Which Foods Cause Vulvodynia Flareups?

Some foods can exacerbate vulvodynia symptoms. Foods high in sugar, yeast, gluten, and dairy may contribute to yeast infections, and sometimes limiting your intake of these foods can help reduce yeast infections [1].

Some women may have allergies or sensitivities to certain foods—like gluten, nuts, or dairy—which can contribute to vulval pain [2]. While further research is needed in this area, some patients have reported a link between celiac disease (gluten intolerance) and vulvodynia [3].

One study published in 2016 linked soy, goat dairy, and gluten to vulvodynia flare ups. Doctors put a 28-year-old woman on an elimination diet, meaning they eliminated a number of foods from her diet then started to reintroduce them one at a time. Foods the researchers tested also included meat, dairy, soy, corn, sugar, artificial sweeteners, and peanuts. Every two weeks, they introduced new foods to the woman's diet and had her report any symptoms. While on the elimination diet, the patient's vulval pain subsided. But the pain returned when she added soy, goat dairy, and gluten back into her diet [4].

Can Supplements Help?

In the above study, researchers found that certain supplements also helped reduce vulvodynia symptoms. In addition to eliminating soy, goat dairy, and gluten, the woman started supplementing her diet with magnesium, vitamin D3, vitamin B12, omega-3, and probiotics. Taking these supplements helped eliminate not only her vulvodynia, but her IBS (irritable bowel syndrome) as well. The woman was still symptom-free six months after the study concluded [4].

Can Probiotics Help?

Probiotics are live microorganisms found in dietary supplements, fermented food, and yogurt. In some cases, probiotics may help women with vulvodynia. For example, they may "help your body maintain a healthy community of microorganisms or help your body's community of microorganisms return to a healthy condition after being disturbed; produce substances that have desirable effects; and influence your body's immune response" [5].

Clinically trialed oral probiotics such as Optibac Probiotics contain 2.3 billion live cultures per capsule. These cultures (which contain Lactobacillus reuteri RC-14 and Lactobacillus rhamnosus GR-1) are designed to help treat and prevent the recurrence of cystitis, thrush, and bacterial vaginosis (BV). You may want to ask your doctor or nutritionist if probiotics are a good option for you.

Are Oxalates Linked to Vulvodynia?

In 1991, an American medical journal reported a link between vulvodynia and oxalate. Foods that are high in oxalate include certain vegetables like rhubarb, beets, and spinach, as well as foods like sweet potatoes, beans, nuts, tofu, and wheat bran. Berries and oranges also contain high amounts of oxalate, as do beverages like coffee, black tea, and soda. Chocolate and foods with soy in them, like soy milk and soy beans, also contain oxalate [6].

As the 1991 report explained, researchers found an abnormally high amount of oxalate in the urine of a woman suffering from vulvodynia. By reducing her oxalate intake and starting her on a calcium citrate supplement, the researchers were able to eliminate the woman's vulval pain. As the levels of oxalate in her urine fell, her symptoms resolved. Because of this report, some people assume that a low-oxalate diet with calcium citrate supplement can help relieve vulvodynia [6].

While it's certainly not worth ruling out altogether, no other studies have supported this conclusion. In fact, researchers have conducted several studies on this subject, but none have been able to prove that oxalate is connected to vulvodynia. As a 2008 study reported: "we saw no association between increasing consumption of various food items high in oxalate content and the risk of vulvodynia" [7].

While these studies haven't found any link between oxalates and vulval pain, they also haven't proven that there is no link. For some women, reducing their oxalate intake and supplementing with calcium citrate may be worth a try.

Making Dietary Changes

In a 2018 study, a 34-year-old pregnant woman was able to reduce vulvodynia symptoms by cutting out dairy, gluten, soy, and processed sugars and taking nutritional supplements [8]. In her own words:

"Changing my diet played an instrumental part in changing my health. I suffered with severe pain, anxiety and depression. Now, I feel almost 100% improved. I no longer eat dairy, gluten, soy or processed sugars. Making the change was extremely hard, especially in social situations. It took me about a year to finally change my eating habits completely. In order for me to make the switch, there were a couple of things I had to do which included: working with a nutritionist who specialized in this, asking family and friends who were closest to me to support me in this change, practicing being kind to myself when I did eat something that was not on my diet, really making a conscious effort to read food labels and educate myself on what I could and could not have, and bringing snacks with me wherever I went, in case I went somewhere that did not have foods that I could eat. The change did not happen overnight. It truly was a lifestyle change—a process. However, it gave me life back. It was hard, but well worth it. I would not be where I am today without making these diet changes. Today, I can instantly tell when I eat something that is not on my diet because I immediately have symptoms flare. In short, the diet was paramount to my healing" [8].

Since the woman was pregnant and in postpartum during the study, autoimmune factors may also have played a role in her recovery, and so we can't be sure exactly how much of that recovery was due to dietary changes. But the study certainly suggests that dietary restrictions and nutritional supplements can help relieve vulvodynia, especially since the patient experienced notable flareups of her symptoms when she consumed gluten, dairy, soy, and sugar—both during her prenatal and postpartum periods. Targeted probiotics and antioxidant supplements may also have played a role in her recovery [8].

Should I Meet with a Functional Nutritionist?

Functional nutrition is about more than simply food. A functional nutritionist can help you plan meals, obtain the right supplements, make lifestyle changes, and learn more about the root causes of your pain.

If you suffer from vulval pain, it can't hurt to meet with a functional nutritionist. While dietary changes may not completely resolve your vulvodynia, there's always a chance they can help relieve it. As the Women's Health Institute states, "a complete functional nutrition assessment and therapeutic recommendations are key strategies for getting to the root cause healing of vulvodynia..." [9].

If you need help finding a functional nutritionist, ask your doctor for a referral, or try the nutrition department at your local hospital or college. You may also be able to ask your insurance company to help you find a nutritionist.

If you live in the US or Canada, you can search online via the Academy of Nutrition and Dietetics (AND), which has a database of nutrition experts at https://www.eatright.org/find-a-nutrition-expert.

Chapter 18

Acupuncture, Vaginal Acupressure, and Manual Trigger Point Therapy for Vulvodynia

Acupuncture

"There are reports of beneficial effects of acupuncture in vulvodynia by switching off the overactive pain fibers" [1].

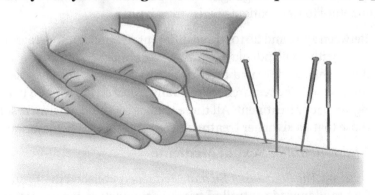

According to the National Institutes of Health (NIH) "Acupuncture is one complementary and alternative medicine therapy used by many patients with vulvodynia; some case reports show that acupuncture may be an effective intervention" [2]. In fact, the

National Institute for Health and Care Excellence (NICE) now includes acupuncture in its guidelines for chronic pain.

How Does Acupuncture Work?

Nerve fibers can transmit pain to the body. By reducing the amplification of nerve fiber transmissions, acupuncture minimizes any pain that stems from these transmissions. This is accomplished by inserting fine, sterile acupuncture needles at acupoints (acupuncture points).

These acupoints may include points from traditional Chinese meridian theory, and points within the pudendal nerve distribution, depending on the practitioner. The needles do not necessarily need to be placed close to the vulva.

You may need several sessions of acupuncture before your pain resolves.

Is Acupuncture Effective for Vulvodynia?

A study published in 2019 found that in a group of 60 women with vulvodynia, acupuncture was the second most frequently used non-drug pain relief strategy after herbal medicine, with 27% of women having used it [3].

In addition, three small but well-conducted and well-reported prospective studies highlight the potential benefits of using acupuncture to treat patients with vulvodynia.

Between 1999 and 2010, three different research groups recruited women with vulvodynia, vulvar vestibulitis, and provoked vestibulodynia; and treated them with five, 10, or 13 weekly sessions of acupuncture. The researchers carefully assessed the women before, during, and after treatment. All three studies reported positive results, but those that used longer treatment courses reported better results.

The Journal of Sexual Medicine

In 2015, *The Journal of Sexual Medicine* published the results of the first randomized controlled trial of acupuncture for women with vulvodynia. According to the results, vulvar pain and painful sexual intercourse "were significantly reduced... and there appeared to be significant improvement in sexual functioning for those receiving acupuncture. Acupuncture did not significantly increase sexual desire, sexual arousal, lubrication, ability to orgasm, or sexual satisfaction in women with vulvodynia" [4].

The researchers concluded that acupuncture is a feasible and worthwhile treatment option for vulvodynia sufferers. Indeed, this small sample alone seemed "to reduce vulvar pain and dyspareunia with an increase in overall sexual function for women with vulvodynia" [4].

The research thus far is positive but limited in terms of the size of the groups studied. Hopefully, further research will be conducted in larger groups of women with vulvodynia.

Should I Try Acupuncture for Vulvodynia?

Currently, the evidence for using acupuncture to treat vulvodynia sufferers is limited. Of course, that doesn't mean that acupuncture can't work for you. If you are interested in trying it, acupuncture is unlikely to do any harm, and could be beneficial.

When performed by qualified practitioners, acupuncture has been shown to be a safe treatment, with minimal adverse effects [5]. We recommend trying at least 10 sessions before making a judgement on whether acupuncture is effective for you.

Acupressure

"An attending nurse or another person must be present and give 'holding' and support to the patient" [6].

How Does Acupressure Work?

Acupressure is a manual therapy treatment used to relieve pain and muscle tension. It is similar to acupuncture in that it uses trigger points, but instead of needles, acupressure is performed with fingers. The practitioner gradually presses their fingers onto specific points, known as trigger points, within muscles and soft tissues, providing pain relief and muscle relaxation. They adjust the amount of pressure to achieve optimal results.

According to a research paper published in *The Scientific World Journal* "Vaginal acupressure is technically the simplest procedure as it corresponds to the explorative phase of the classic pelvic examination, except that the purpose of the digital penetration is treatment and not examination" [6].

During a vaginal acupressure session, an experienced physician can normally locate all the necessary organs. They "penetrate the vagina with one or two fingers and presses systematically on the sore and tense areas in the pelvis... The position of the physician's hand must be so that only the structures that need to be touched are contacted. It is important that the clitoris is not touched unintentionally" [6].

This procedure is similar to "the same explorative part of the standard pelvic examination by a gynecologist, but in this case done so slowly that the woman can feel the emotions held by the different tissues contacted by the finger of the physician" [4].

Acupressure treatment can be conducted at the same time as a pelvic examination, since broadly speaking, there is an element of acupressure in a pelvic examination. During an acupressure session, you may experience emotionally painful, unpleasant feelings; but your gynecologist or physician will likely prepare you for these sensations ahead of time [6].

Ethical Standards

Before booking a vaginal acupuncture appointment, make sure that the treatment complies with your country's medical authority's ethical standards. While a standard pelvic examination can be conducted by most physicians after they have completed their general medical training, vaginal acupressure can only be practiced by a physician who has undergone substantial training and supervision in acupressure techniques [6].

Are There Any Adverse-Effects?

Potential negative side effects may include feeling sore in some of the areas where the acupressure has been applied. You may also experience old, painful, pent-up thoughts resurfacing, which can lead to depression. But note that this is actually a good thing, as it can help you let go, rid yourself of this deep-seated negativity, and heal your body. Any discomfort from the pressure points should dissipate within a short period of time [6].

Is Acupressure Effective for Vulvodynia?

Acupressure via the vagina could be a valuable therapy for improving vulvodynia. But to confirm this theory, further research is needed. Traditional acupressure techniques through the vagina have been developed and tested at the Copenhagen Research Clinic for Holistic Medicine. This treatment was presented at the Second International Conference on Holistic Health in Oslo, Norway, in 2005 [6].

Personalized Treatment

Your personal circumstances are of prime importance when acupressure via the vagina is administered. For example, if you suffer from long-term pain in the pelvis or sexual organs (primary vulvodynia), or a long-term bladder infection, then the treatment is given differently.

"If the physician believes several methods to be equally efficient, they should always tell the patient about the alternative treatments and respect the patient's choice" [6].

Manual Trigger Point Therapy

The American College of Obstetricians and Gynecologists promote a type of massage known as trigger point therapy. In this case, a trigger point refers to a small area of muscle which is extremely contracted. Nearby areas can also be painful, due to the sensation which emanates from a trigger point.

This form of therapy, much like the acupressure procedure described above, involves massaging the affected soft tissue to relax the tight muscle areas. In the college's words "a combination of an anesthetic drug and a steroid can also be injected into the trigger point to provide relief" [7].

Chapter 19

TENS for Vulvodynia

"TENS constitutes a feasible and beneficial addition to multidimensional treatment for therapy-resistant Provoked Vestibulodynia" [1].

What Is TENS?

In transcutaneous electrical nerve stimulation (TENS), a non-invasive electrical nerve stimulator sends low-voltage electrical pulses through the skin to the underlying nerves. TENS has few adverse effects and can be applied in several areas, including:

- Around the source of the pain
- To acupuncture points near the pain
- To a dermatome (an area of the skin supplied by nerves from a single spinal root) via electrodes
- Intra-vaginally via a vaginal probe

It's best to try different electrode positions until you find the most comfortable, effective position for you.

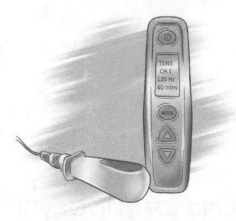

How Does It Work?

There are two main theories about how TENS works.

Theory 1. The electric current excites the nerve cells that block the transmission of pain signals, thus altering the sufferer's perception of pain.

Theory 2. Stimulating the nerves raises the level of the body's natural pain-killing chemicals (endorphins), which work to block the sufferer's sense of pain.

The level of stimulation generated by the device determines which nerve fibres are stimulated, thus enabling the user to experience some degree of pain relief. In the case of vulvodynia sufferers, pulsed currents are delivered via TENS electrodes or a TENS vaginal probe.

"High frequency and low frequency TENS activate different opioid receptors. Both applications have been shown to provide analgesia specifically when applied at a strong, non-painful intensity. High frequency TENS may be more effective for people taking opioids" [4].

What Does the Research Say?

One randomized controlled trial compared a vaginal TENS probe against a sham device (placebo or device with no therapeutic value). The researchers used a TENS unit to treat participants' vestibulodynia two times a week for 10 weeks. "Pain scores, dyspareunia and overall sexual functioning were significantly improved in the active arm compared to placebo" [1].

Another randomized controlled trial, entitled "Vaginal diazepam plus transcutaneous electrical nerve stimulation to treat vestibulodynia," [5] assessed the effectiveness of combining vaginal diazepam with TENS in the treatment of vestibulodynia. The researchers concluded that "the study provided indications that vaginal diazepam plus TENS is useful to improve pain and pelvic floor muscle (PFM) instability in women with vestibulodynia" [5].

Other studies suggests that "since vestibulodynia is considered to belong to chronic pain syndromes, a TENS approach might be reasonable; TENS is of significant benefit in the management of vestibulodynia, at least on a relatively short-term basis" [6]. In other words, TENS has helped provide relief for some vulvodynia and vestibulodynia sufferers.

Vulvar Pain, Sexual Functioning, and Sexually Related Distress

The Journal for Sexual Medicine published promising research on these very important subjects. The scientists summarised that "the addition of self-administered TENS to multidimensional treatment significantly reduced the level of vulvar pain and the need for vestibulectomy. The long-term effect was stable. These results support the hypothesis that TENS constitutes a feasible and beneficial addition to multidimensional treatment for therapy-resistant provoked vestibulodynia" [1].

Based on the research, TENS is emerging as a potentially effective treatment for women with vulvodynia. If you are interested in trying it yourself, ask your doctor or clinician for more information.

Chapter 20

Diaphragmatic Breathing and Yoga

Do You Have Poor Posture?

With so many people doing sedentary work, not to mention all the hours we spend looking at a screen, it's not surprising that we spend far too much of our lives sitting down. Unfortunately, this means that our transverse abdominus muscles (the muscles that help prevent back pain), may be weak.

"This can be linked to pelvic floor problems. For example, if we collapse our chest while sitting, we end up with a 'C-curve' in the spine. This makes it challenging to take a deep breath, and consequently, the muscles of the pelvic floor don't receive the gentle 'exercise' they need, stretching and contracting with every breath in and out" [2].

Everything in the body is connected, and one of the most effective ways to take care of the pelvic floor is to practice diaphragmatic breathing [2].

What is Diaphragmatic Breathing?

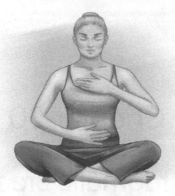

Diaphragmatic breathing (deep breathing or belly breathing) refers to a method of deep breathing that involves the diaphragm, a dome-shaped muscle at the bottom of the rib cage. Diaphragmatic breathing offers several excellent benefits, including helping you relax, which is highly beneficial for women suffering from vulvodynia; and reducing the detrimental effects of the stress hormone cortisol [1].

"Breathing into your belly may seem like a convenient metaphor for active and engaged breathing, but the breath does literally affect the muscles of the abdomen and the pelvic floor. A deep breath that goes into the abdomen benefits the pelvic floor in many ways" [2].

When you breathe in, your diaphragm contracts and moves downward. This causes your lungs to enlarge, generating negative pressure which propels air in through your nose and mouth until your lungs fill up with air. When you breathe out, the muscles in your diaphragm relax and move upwards, sending air out of your lungs via your breath [1].

Re-Learning the Correct Way to Breathe

"A healthy pelvic floor stretches as we breathe in and contracts slightly as the breath goes up and out" [2].

With so much stress negatively affecting you 24/7, the carefree breathing that you once enjoyed as a child may have given way to shallow breathing that only uses the chest. Stress, poor posture, tight clothing, and other scenarios that weaken the muscles can all contribute to chest breathing.

Specialists state that "retraining ourselves to breathe with our bellies can help shallow breathers rely less on their chests, and more on their diaphragms as they move their bellies out to inhale and in to exhale" [1].

There's a simple technique you can use to practice diaphragmatic breathing, which we'll discuss below. While it may take time to master, the benefits will be well worth it.

If you have a lung condition, consult your medical practitioner before attempting any breathing exercises [1].

"Diaphragmatic breathing allows us the opportunity to stretch the pelvic floor throughout the day and can even be performed during sex to decrease pain" [1].

How to Practice Diaphragmatic Breathing

1. Find a Quiet Place and a Good Posture

Choose a quiet place where you can sit or lie down comfortably. You can either lie on your back, sit cross-legged on the floor, or sit in a chair.

If you're sitting, be sure to relax your shoulders, neck, and head muscles. If you're in a chair, bend your knees and place your feet on the floor. While you don't need to sit as straight as a board, try not to slouch.

If you choose to lie down, you may bend your knees if it's comfortable for you, or stretch them out straight. You may also want to put a small pillow under your head [1].

2. Put One Hand on Your Upper Chest

Place one hand on your upper chest. Keep this hand still throughout the exercise [1].

3. Put the Other Hand Under Your Ribcage

Place your other hand under your ribcage, just above your navel (your belly button). This will enable you to feel your diaphragm moving as you breathe [1].

4. Breath in Through Your Nose

Now breathe in slowly through your nose for five seconds. As the air travels in through your nose, you should feel your belly rise beneath your hand.

Do not push or force your abdominal muscles outwards, and don't clench your muscles to try and force the lower part of your belly out. Instead, let your breath do the work.

Keep the hand on your chest relatively still. You should feel your rib cage and abdomen slowly expanding beneath your other hand, and then gently returning to their resting state [1].

5. Breathe Out Through Your Mouth

Now breath out slowly for five seconds through your mouth, keeping your lips slightly pursed. As you do so, allow your belly to relax. The hand on your belly should fall inwards towards your spine.

Do not clench or squeeze your muscles to force your stomach inward. Keep the hand on your chest relatively still [1].

After mastering this technique, perform it one to four times per day, over a period of five to 10 minutes. If you have a condition which makes this practice difficult for you, adjust to meet your individual circumstances.

Yoga

Yoga has been around for thousands of years and can benefit both the mind and body. It empowers you with the chance to reflect internally and to practice slow, mindful breathing and movements. No matter your age or flexibility, you can still practice yoga, which encourages working at your own level and pace. Even just doing limited poses and breathing exercises can be extremely beneficial, and you do not need to become an expert! [3]

Yoga can help improve pelvic health and breathing, both of which can be helpful for relieving vulvodynia symptoms. But there's another benefit as well.

In the case of "women recovering from trauma, including medical trauma of being under-diagnosed or mismanaged, anxiety is usually present. When you have another tool in your toolbox (such as yoga), to manage stress and anxiety caused by pelvic health concerns, you are empowered to take control of your body and retrain your brain" [3].

Let's look at some yoga poses that can help you practice breathing and relieve anxiety and vulvodynia symptoms. For the following exercises, you will need a yoga or floor mat. Alternately, you can perform these exercises on a carpet or towel, but a yoga mat will give you the best results.

Child's Pose

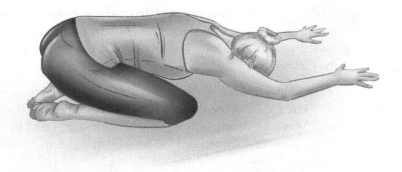

This popular yoga pose is a great pelvic floor stretch. First, go into a kneeling position on your mat, with your toes together and your knees wide apart. If kneeling is painful for you, try placing a rolled-up blanket or towel under your knees [4].

Now, still kneeling, sit up with your back straight. Gently move your head toward the ground and extend your arms on the floor in front of you, as if reaching forward. If this is too difficult for your back, hips, or knees, place your forearms on the floor in front of you and rest your head in your arms [4].

As soon as you are comfortably in this position, start to take large, slow breaths. On the inhale, you might experience a mild drop through your pelvic floor, and on the exhale, you might feel a mild rise.

Continue breathing in Child's Pose for anywhere from 30 seconds to several minutes [4].

Happy Baby Pose

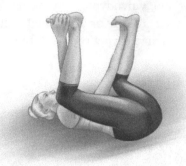

This much-loved yoga pose involves lying comfortably on your back on top of your mat. Inhale deeply, then exhale, drawing your knees up toward your underarms, keeping your knees and feet wide apart (see the picture below).

Now, either hold onto the outside of your feet with your hands, or if this is not comfortable, place them on your knees or shins. If you want to, you can even try lifting your feet above your knees, parallel to the ground (although this should not be held for long). Once you've reached your desired position, breathe slowly in and out [4].

One of the nicest things about the Happy Baby Pose is that you can intensify it by gently rocking your hips backwards and forwards, unbending and bending your lower back against the ground until you feel comfortable.

When you inhale, you might experience the same soft drop that you felt in Child's Pose. On the exhale, you may feel the same soft rise. Inhale and exhale in this position for a minimum of 30 seconds, or longer if you feel comfortable doing so [4].

How Often Should I Do These Yoga Poses?

For best results, repeat the Happy Baby and Child's Pose exercises a minimum of two to three times daily, for 30 seconds to several minutes each [4]. If you need help figuring out how to do these poses, you can find instructional yoga videos online.

Chapter 21

Psychological Treatments for Vulvodynia

Back at the beginning of this book, we debunked the myth that sexual abuse can cause vulvodynia. While that remains true, traumatic experiences like abuse may increase your risk of developing vulvodynia by heightening your sensitivity to pain. And while it's also true that vulvodynia is not simply "all in your mind," the pain and stress of vulvodynia can cause you further pain. These facts are important to keep in mind as you read this chapter. At no point should you feel that vulvodynia is your fault, that it's something you're imagining, or that you could avoid it entirely by just being less anxious. Having said that, let's look at the relationship between psychological stressors and vulvodynia.

"A history of anxiety disorders and major depression is 11 and 4 times more prevalent, respectively, in women with PVD compared to non-afflicted women" [1].

12% of women are likely to experience PVD (provoked vestibulodynia) during their lifetime, and PVD is the most enduring reason for the pain pre-menopausal women experience (dyspareunia) during sexual intercourse [2].

"Reductions in sexual desire and arousal and decreased frequency of intercourse are common in women with PVD" [1].

When sexual intercourse is extremely painful or even impossible, as for PVD sufferers, it can be damaging psychologically. Particularly, it may affect the sufferer's self-esteem and emotional well-being; and it can damage intimate relationships [2].

But the good news is, you don't have to continue suffering. If PVD or vulvodynia is affecting your relationships and emotional health, you have options. In this chapter, we'll look at the research on using psychological therapy for vulvodynia, and discuss possible psychological treatment options.

Why Choose Psychological Treatments for PVD?

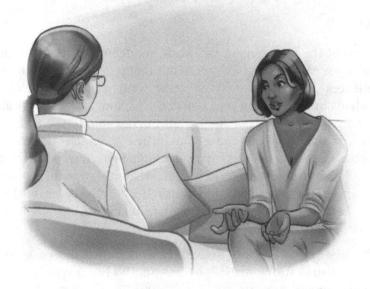

Because PVD medication can bring negative side effects, many practitioners are now choosing to focus instead on psychological treatments. According to a 2016 study published in the *Journal of Clinical Psychology* "Psychological treatments for PVD have the advantage of targeting both the experience of pain and its many psychosexual consequences, such as reduced desire and arousal" [2]. The goal of such treatments is not just to allow you to have sex again, but to restore your pleasure by removing painful associations and discomfort from sexual activities.

What Does the Research Say?

PVD sufferers report "lower levels of pleasure during sexual activity and less success in reaching orgasm. In addition to a decrease in sexual pleasure during penetrative sex, women with genital pain often describe diminished sexual desire for an array of non-penetrative activities" [1]. Research also indicates that women who experience genital pain have greater difficulty managing intimate relationships [1].

These women may feel "discomfort with their sexual self, often reporting a general sense of detachment from their sexuality. It has been repeatedly shown that women with genital pain experience negative feelings toward erotic stimuli, negative emotions during sexual activity, a more negative sexual self-view, and more negative attitudes toward sexuality" [1].

Combating these feelings can help you regain control of your intimate relationships and start enjoying your sexual experiences instead of dreading them. Again, it's worth noting that the goal of treatment is not simply to satisfy your partner's desire for sexual activity, but to give you pleasure and improve the way you view yourself and your relationships.

Depression, Stress, and Anxiety

While PVD is not simply a mental or emotional condition, it does have an interesting relationship with your emotional and mental health.

Research indicates that depression, stress, and anxiety can "act as vulnerabilities to the development of PVD, and not simply a consequence of experiencing it and that there is a reciprocal relationship. Anxiety may represent an important factor in the occurrence of PVD" [1].

Further, women who experience PVD may develop anxiety as a result, and anxiety and harm avoidance can serve to heighten pain during intercourse [1].

"Greater pain sensitivity and anxiety potentially lead to the avoidance of intercourse by overestimating the level of potential harm" [1].

PVD can be a vicious cycle. The effects of PVD can serve to heighten your stress and mood symptoms, and these symptoms can trigger more painful experiences. Because you have experienced intense pain, you are more likely than others to go out of your way to avoid experiencing that pain again. You are also more likely to experience psychological distress as real physical pain, and more likely to be pre-occupied with physical sensations. You may also experience heightened fear that others will see you in a negative light, and may even develop dislike toward yourself [1].

In addition to this, stress-generated, neuroendocrine interactions (between the endocrine system and the nervous system) "have been linked to the proliferation of pain receptor cells along the sensory nerve endings of vestibular tissue in women with PVD, [and] stimulation of these cells activates chronic inflammation, nerve hypersensitivity, and pain" [1].

In other words, when you experience stress, it can affect your hormone and nervous system interactions, causing rapid growth of pain receptor cells in the vagina. When these receptor cells get chronically inflamed, it causes hypersensitivity and pain. Unfortunately, this means that stressing about your pain can potentially cause you more pain. For precisely this reason, it's important to learn how to manage your pain and stress psychologically.

Psychological States Influence Your Sensitivity to Pain

Psychological distress and pain sensitivity "increases the risk for pain moving from being acute, to chronic. Chronic pain is highly associated with anxiety and depression, and vice versa" [6]. Research suggests that traumatic childhood experiences such as abuse, being fearful of abuse, and social trauma (e.g., lack of support, exclusion, and bullying), are also risk factors for PVD and long-term pain [6].

In addition to this, women who have had Post Traumatic Stress Disorder (PTSD) are at risk of developing PVD; in fact, their risk is two to three times higher than the norm. Co-occurring long-term pain and PTSD are linked to pain disability and increased levels of pain. Pain catastrophizing (excessive pain worries) is also a firmly established risk factor for elevated pain perception. This includes not being able to inhibit pain-related fears, magnification of the pain's negative effects, anxious preoccupation with pain, and a sense of helplessness when experiencing pain [6].

Psychosexual Therapy

In this popular counseling approach, a therapist can help assess your sexual functioning and provide information, education, and details about support groups for both couples and individuals. This approach is very beneficial for some women, as it combines sexual and psychological therapy, considering both psychological and somatic (body) issues and symptoms [1].

The British Society for the Study of Vulval Disease recommends "desensitization of the vulva for allodynia (resulting from a stimulus which would not usually provoke pain), with psychosexual and physical therapy as first-line techniques" [1]. In other words, a combination of physical and psychological therapy is recommended, this is known as psychosexual therapy.

In psychosexual therapy, a registered psychologist or psychotherapist will help you work through various strategies to manage your pain more effectively, over the course of several appointments. They may help you understand the complex pain system and the reciprocal relationships between pain and mood, teaching you CBT strategies and mindfulness (which we'll discuss later in this chapter). You may also learn pacing and attention strategies that you can use to prevent pain wind-up (an increase in pain intensity over time). If appropriate, you may want to attend some of these appointments with your sexual partner so you can work through any communication and expectation issues under the guidance of your therapist.

Cognitive Behavioral Therapy (CBT)

"CBT is considered a mainstay of treatment for chronic pain, and consistently shows moderate to high efficacy rates in the treatment of PVD, ranging from 35% to 85%" [1].

CBT is short for cognitive behavioral therapy. The word "cognitive" refers to thinking, or conscious mental processes. Currently "CBT represents one of the most popular first-line psychological interventions for PVD. Mindfulness has been increasingly used alongside, or instead of CBT with respect to chronic pain disorders, and more recently in women with PVD" [2].

Since CBT and mindfulness have proven so effective for treating PVD, let's look at both these strategies in greater detail.

How Does CBT Work?

When used for PVD, CBT focuses on addressing "maladaptive pain-related cognitions, change-oriented psycho-education, and behavioral interventions, such as specific pain relevant coping and self-management skills" [1].

CBT helps to change the way you think about pain, which enables your mind and body to better cope. CBT is based on the understanding that long-term genital pain negatively affects your psychological, sexual, and relational health [1]. The way you think about your pain can impact how you respond when the pain comes, and as we discussed earlier, this can become a vicious cycle that only increases your distress and pain and decreases your quality of life. By changing the way you adapt and respond to pain, CBT can help improve general sexual dysfunction, decrease your fear of pain, and reduce vulvar pain.

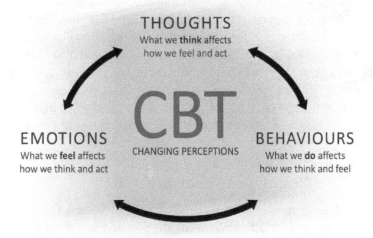

What Does the Research Say?

Research indicates that CBT indirectly reduces women's symptoms of PVD by combating stress. CBT "has been found to

exacerbate one's vulnerability to developing pain syndromes; [and] dysregulate pain sensitivity" [1]. In other words, CBT can in fact be helpful for treating painful and distressing symptoms of PVD, because it enables you to better manage the stress associated with these symptoms.

A Three-Month Trial

In 2007, a three-month trial examined how CBT works to reduce chronic vaginismus (a painful muscle spasm in the PFM). Researchers randomly assigned the participants to two groups: a control group (group that did not receive treatment) and a CBT group. The results were very promising "compared to controls, women in the CBT group reported a higher frequency of intercourse, a decrease in fear of penetrative sex, and more successful non-coital penetrative behavior from pre- to post-treatment" [1]. The researchers concluded that "CBT techniques, namely, gradual exposure exercises aimed at reducing avoidance behavior and fear of penetration, represent a viable treatment for lifelong vaginismus" [1].

Two Randomized Controlled Trials

A randomized control trial (RCT) is a clinical study in which participants are chosen at random to receive one of a number of different treatments. Those treatments may include a placebo (often referred to as a sugar pill), a standard practice, or no intervention at all [3]. In a standard randomized control trial, one group receives this type of "treatment," while the other receives the treatment type being tested. Researchers can them measure the results of the two groups against each other.

Two randomized control studies from the last fifteen years evaluated how effective CBT is for PVD. In one of the studies, led by Bergeron et al., participants were randomly placed into one of three groups: vestibulectomy (the surgical removal of the posterior hymen and anterior and posterior vestibule mucosa), pelvic floor biofeedback, or CBT.

In the CBT group, participants received 10 group sessions of CBT. The results showed "a reduction in pain intensity, significantly improved psychological adjustment, and improved sexual function. Participants from all three groups reported significant reductions in pain, with vestibulectomy resulting in the greatest pain reduction

(47%–70%), followed by CBT (21%–38%), and biofeedback (19%–35%)" [1].

All three treatments improved the participants' sexual function, and at a two-and-a-half-year follow-up, all the improvements remained steady. Of course, the most effective treatment option in this study was vestibulectomy. But this surgery is not risk-free, and many women prefer a less invasive treatment option [1].

In the other randomized clinical trial, women with provoked vulvodynia tested a personalized 10-week CBT program against supportive psychotherapy, which is much less active and strategic. Both options "significantly improved pain severity, sexual function, and psychological function. However, relative to women in the supportive psychotherapy group, participants in the CBT group reported significantly greater treatment gains, including greater improvements in overall sexual function and pain severity ratings during gynecological examination" [1]. These findings remained the same at a follow-up session a year later [1].

Based on the results, the researchers hypothesized that CBT strategies "were more beneficial in mitigating pain provoked by touch and enhancing sexual function, in contrast to a talk therapy, which lacks behavioral interventions" [1].

The women in the CBT group "also reported greater treatment satisfaction; as pain severity ratings and overall sexual function were the only measures significantly correlated with treatment satisfaction" [1]. Pain severity and sexual function may be the most important factors in whether a PVD patient is satisfied with the results of her treatment [1].

To some extent at least, these two trials support using CBT for PVD sufferers. Indeed, the results "suggest that the directive approach of CBT represents a promising avenue toward yielding better outcomes and greater treatment satisfaction compared to a less directive approach" [1].

Mindfulness

"Mindfulness has been shown to provide physical pain relief and reduce pain-related brain activity, as well as

lessening the devastating emotional and functional impairments associated with PVD" [1].

Mindfulness is similar to meditation, but in this context, mindfulness is not associated with any religious practice. Instead, it's simply about being aware of your thoughts, feelings, and experiences. Mindfulness means being present in the moment, without judging or trying to change your thoughts and feelings.

It has been described as a state of "mental focus that emphasizes acceptance and awareness of the present moment without judgment or evaluation. This state of mind or style of thinking can be thought of as a personal trait or as a cognitive skill that can be exercised and improved upon over time" [1].

To put it a little differently, mindfulness is "an intentional shift toward observing one's present experience without altering it, where thoughts freely enter conscious awareness and are then let go with the absence of any emotional attachment or reaction" [1]. Due to its promising association with positive sexual outcomes, psychological health, and emotional well-being, mindfulness has become increasingly popular [1].

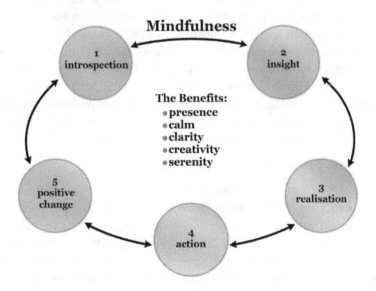

"Despite the compelling rationale, there is a dearth of published data applying mindfulness to the treatment of PVD" [1].

Over the last 10 years or so, mindfulness has become more and more popular for managing long-term pain disorders. Sometimes mindfulness is used in conjunction with CBT, but sometimes it's used alone. A 2011 meta-analysis study compared CBT to mindfulness-based therapy and determined that "mindfulness approaches represent a viable alternative to CBT, with particular efficacy for individuals who had found CBT less helpful" [1].

A meta-analysis study is a statistical process that combines data from multiple studies. When the effect of the treatment (or effect size) is consistent in each study, this form of analysis helps to identify this common effect [4].

"Research has linked low mindfulness to hypervigilance of pain as well as pain catastrophizing, both of which are characteristic of women with PVD" [1].

Whereas CBT uses a change-oriented approach, mindfulness-based therapy uses an acceptance-based approach. This can work well for treating chronic pain conditions and emotional stress [1]. Research conducted in the last ten years compared the effectiveness of a short CBT program with a MBT (mindfulness-based therapy) intervention for individuals with sexual distress and a history of childhood sexual abuse. The results showed that both treatments "led to a significant decrease in sexual distress. Women in the MBT group also experienced a significantly greater increase in concordance (i.e. agreement) between personal report and physical changes experienced in sexual arousal, compared to the CBT group" [1].

Stress Awareness Via Mindfulness

Like CBT, mindfulness can give you more control over how you respond to pain. This may be because mindfulness helps combat central sensitization, or your body's intensifying response to pain that occurs repeatedly over time. It may also help with neuroendocrine interactions (the relationship between your endocrine and nervous systems) and skin pathophysiology (disordered skin processes due to injury or disease) [1]. In layman's terms, mindfulness brings many benefits to both the mind and body because it allows you to control, in some measure, how you react to pain and other sensations.

"Mindfulness has been linked to a host of improved sexual outcomes, including enhanced sexual desire, vaginal lubrication, body esteem, and sexual satisfaction, as well as reducing sexual distress and anxiety" [1].

The emotional pain of PVD sufferers can be "uncoupled from the associated physical sensation of pain. This mindful separation of emotions from physical pain cultivates awareness of responses that exacerbate pain, such as fearful anticipation" [1]. Mindfulness empowers you to re-evaluate your response to the pain you feel [1]. This helps you notice that your thoughts, emotions, and responses are not necessarily dependent on your pain.

Being in the Now

"Studies show that mindfulness techniques can facilitate pain relief and improve both the functional and emotional elements of chronic pain" [1].

Mindfulness offers a promising pathway toward reducing your pain by shifting your focus to the here and now. One study showed "significant improvements in catastrophizing after a 10-week mindfulness intervention for chronic pain management" [1]. If you can increase your ability to consciously center your attention on the present, it may help you kick the habit of catastrophizing (imagining the worst possible scenario) or anticipating pain [1].

Being Non-Judgmental

Practicing mindfulness helps you be non-judgmental and accepting. This is especially important for PVD sufferers, as PVD can lead to feelings of low self-acceptance and high self-criticism. In fact, encouraging self-acceptance and discouraging negative thoughts about yourself may be the most important way mindfulness can help to reduce your symptoms. When you lower your self-criticism, you reduce the impact of stress on your body. And as we've seen already, reducing your stress and anxiety can go a long way toward helping you heal.

Being Accepting

Acceptance is about living well with pain but not passively allowing it. In other words, it's a "willingness to continue to actively experience pain, along with related thoughts and feelings" [1]. This may help you become more self-compassionate, encouraging you to face and acknowledge your emotional response to pain in a non-judgmental way. According to one source, "mindfulness can significantly improve pain self-efficacy and reduce genital pain vigilance and awareness in women with PVD" [1].

But mindfulness does more than just help you live with pain; it also increases your capacity for pleasure. When you think in an aware, non-judgmental way over time, you can become more in tune with your sexual self. A short mindfulness-based psychoeducational intervention (an approach that combines counseling, education, and other supportive methods) determined that mindfulness strategies "significantly improved sexual desire and reduced sexual distress for women suffering from sexual desire and/or sexual arousal disorder" [1]. Mindfulness can also help you recognize and dismiss distracting thoughts that may interrupt your enjoyment of sex [1].

Even in studies where women did not experience a literal physiological change in their sexual response, they were able to improve their perception of that sexual response. Our minds have a strong relationship with our bodies and gaining control over our thoughts and feelings can significantly affect how we experience pain and other sensations.

Yoga and Meditation for Mindfulness

One study from the last 10 years examined the consequences of physical activity on sexuality. The results showed that those "who consistently practiced yoga, or another activity involving a mindfulness component, reported more sexual desire and had higher levels of sexual awareness than individuals who engaged in physical activity lacking in mindfulness" [1].

Basic yoga, which includes meditation, can help you practice mindfulness. You may want to attend regular local classes at a gym or other facility, or sign up for several sessions with a friend, as this is more likely to increase your attendance. Or, if you prefer, you can search YouTube for beginner yoga videos that focus on meditation. Try looking up "beginner yoga videos meditation" or something similar.

There are also many apps you can use to practice mindfulness, or you might try contacting a psychologist, as they are usually trained in how to teach and assist mindfulness.

How Many Sessions of Mindfulness Therapy Will I Need?

While research shows that just four sessions of mindfulness-based therapy can help improve sexual symptoms, longer interventions may offer a higher payoff. It can be hard to do regular practice at home, so attending more sessions might help you gain a greater grasp of mindfulness techniques. Research undertaken by Brotto et al., in 2013 noted that "several women communicated regret for not having prioritized regular skill practice after program completion" [1].

Booking a refresher session or follow-up can help you maintain the progress you've worked for and can also help with problem-solving when new challenges arise. Everyone is different of course, but with individual therapy, close collaboration, and open communication with your psychologist or therapist, you can tailor your sessions to your specific needs.

Using Dilators for Mindfulness

"Mindfulness dilator insertion combines the act of using vaginal inserts with an enhanced emotional awareness, thus lessening feelings of obligation, disassociation, and resentment" [1].

If you want to work toward penetration in sex, a dilator may help you. Dilator therapy involves deep muscle relaxation and the slow insertion of a finger or dilator into the vagina. The goal of this is to lessen your fear and anxiety of penetration, feelings that can be caused by vulvar pain. Of course, the ultimate goal is not just to allow for penetration, but to encourage you to feel more independent and in control of your own body. Dilator therapy in combination with mindfulness can provide a self-governing and uplifting experience that helps unify your mind and body [1].

Mindfulness-Based Cognitive Behavioral Therapy (MBCT)

A mindfulness-based cognitive therapy (MBCT) review in 2012 highlighted MBCT's success in treating mood and anxiety disorders, looking especially at the difference between traditional CBT and MBCT. The reviewers concluded that "CBT promotes a new way of looking at pain, while MBCT encourages a new way of being with pain. Where CBT centers on distinguishing unhelpful thoughts from helpful ones, MBCT aims to identify thoughts as simply normal mental events as opposed to statements of fact" [1].

"MBCT research has highlighted its utility and benefits for treating women with PVD, as well as conditions that are commonly comorbid with PVD, such as depression and anxiety" [1].

Due to the recognized success of CBT, and the wealth of research on mindfulness-based therapies for sexual dysfunction and long-term pain, "an MBCT approach may represent a particularly beneficial approach for treating women with PVD" [1].

CBT and mindfulness can be complimentary therapeutic processes, working together to adjust your experience of pain. Using mindfulness, you can be more aware of negative, unhelpful thoughts. Using CBT, you can then change your response to those thoughts. After a while, you will be able to see your unwelcome emotions and thoughts as temporary things that come and go, not facts that define you. This means that as time passes, you will have less of a need to actively challenge your disturbing thoughts. Instead, you will simply see them drifting in and out of your mind [1].

Think of Pain as a Fellow Journeyman

"Both CBT and mindfulness work to alleviate future-oriented stress and improve co-morbid anxiety and depression through relatively distinct means that together may prove to be particularly efficacious" [1].

CBT and mindfulness combined can also help alleviate anxiety about your pain. For example, if you view the pain not as a cause of trauma but as a fellow journeyman (or woman), you may be able to better deal with it [1].

Avoid Goal-Oriented Language

MCBT encourages you to develop a new perception of sex. Instead of seeing it as a goal or accomplishment, think of it as a meaningful act or experience. Avoid goal-oriented language when thinking or talking about sex [1].

Restoring Sexual Function

Research shows that MBCT can help restore sexual function to women who either suffer or do not suffer pain. CBT encourages you not to avoid sex simply because you believe it will be painful. Of course, if sex causes you intense pain, you may need to take a break from sex while you seek treatment. But at the same time, avoiding sex for a significant period of time can only heighten your trauma associated with it. Instead, try to remember the pleasure you used to associate with sex, and anticipate having a good experience. Take any steps you can to limit pain during intercourse so that it will not be a traumatic experience [1].

More Positive Research

In 2016, Brotto et al., looked at the benefits of attending a mindfulness-based group therapy for PVD sufferers. This therapy, which ran for four sessions, focused on developing mindfulness and meditation skills, as well as teaching and discussing cognitive theory and the practice of various cognitive behavioral skills [1].

After the therapy, the participants experienced substantial improvements in mood and self-esteem, and reductions in sex-related distress, skin sensitivity, pain worries, and over attending to the pain. At follow-up, these findings were still in effect, and some had even improved further. The study uncovered no changes in dyspareunia, but this could be because few of the women engaged in penetrative sex during the length of the study [1].

The women said they felt less isolated and more "normal" because of the therapy, their shared experience, and the group's feeling of community. "All women reported improvements in psychological outcomes as a result of treatment, specifically with respect to lower rates of depression and anxiety, greater self-esteem and self-confidence, excitement and optimism for the future, and an enhanced inclination for positive thinking and acceptance" [1].

The Importance of Psychoeducation

"Prior research demonstrates that education alone can improve PVD symptoms" [1].

In the above study, researchers noted that a basic aspect of MBCT and CBT is psychoeducation (mental health education), which "played a key role in normalizing the participants' perception of their condition" [1]. When women understand that PVD is an intricate medical condition capable of affecting both their mind and body, they are more willing to try psychological therapy for managing their condition. It's likely that in this study, the women's development of CBT and mindfulness skills helped improve the outcome of their treatment [1].

The Benefits of a Multidisciplinary Approach

Given all the information, it makes sense to take a multifaceted approach, combining MBCT and other treatment methods to provide a higher benefit. A 2012 qualitative study showed that "a multidisciplinary vulvodynia program that incorporated pelvic floor physiotherapy, education, and medical management alongside three two-hour sessions of MBCT could be beneficial" [1].

Flexibility in regards to treatment is also possible. For example, MBCT for provoked vulvodynia could be given to patients as an online intervention, with the use of text rather than verbal dialogue, and audio recordings of mindfulness techniques instead of in-person led meditations [1]. This would be ideal for women who for whatever reason, find it difficult to attend regular face-to-face sessions; moreover, it offers the flexibility to be used any day, at any time.

Have Patience

Although the approaches discussed in this chapter can be highly beneficial, remember that psychological progress rarely happens all at once. Obstacles along the way simply represent learning opportunities and problems you can solve. Mindfulness for vulvar pain "emphasizes self-acceptance and letting go of the pressure for change, it is important to highlight the significance of accepting where [you] are at and exercising self-compassion in terms of working within one's availability" [1]. So have patience and grace with yourself as you begin your journey toward recovery.

How Can I Find a CBT or Mindfulness Therapist?

Finding a therapist can be confusing. If you want to practice the approaches in this chapter, then ideally, you're looking for a therapist experienced in psychosexual work, with training or accreditation in CBT and mindfulness. If possible, ask your doctor or clinician for a referral to a CBT or mindfulness therapist. You may get a referral to a local sexual functioning service, where you can find medical and psychological practitioners, but sometimes these services have limited availability.

Alternately, you may be able to find a therapist by searching online. In the US, try the following sites:

- Association for Behavioral and Cognitive Therapies (ABCT): findcbt.org

- American Board of Professional Psychology (ABPP): www.abpp.org

- Academy of Cognitive and Behavioral Therapies (A-CBT): www.academyofct.org

- In the UK, try these sites:

- College of Sexual and Relational Therapists (COSRT): www.cosrt.org.uk

- British Association of Behavioral and Cognitive Psychotherapists (BABCP) has a register of accredited CBT practitioners; find one with psycho-sexual experience: www.babcp.com/Public/Accessing-CBT.aspx

- You can also find online mindfulness resources at:

- Mindful: www.mindful.org/meditation/mindfulness-getting-started/

- Be Mindful: www.bemindful.com (This includes access to a free online mindfulness course.)

- Finally, if you're looking for a book on mindfulness and sex, try:

- Better Sex through Mindfulness: How Women Can Cultivate Desire by Lori A. Brotto, PhD (Published in 2018 by Greystone Book

Chapter 22

Surgical Intervention for Vulvodynia

"Vestibulectomy has always been a controversial treatment, as to many doctors and patients, it seems a drastic step" [1].

Excision of painful skin from the vulvar vestibule was first described in 1983. Since that time, many medical publications have highlighted the benefits of this surgical intervention, but only a small number of gynaecologists specialize in it. To find out if you are a suitable candidate, you will need to talk to a surgeon who has experience with this treatment [2].

What Does the Procedure Entail?

A vestibulectomy is the most common surgical procedure for vulvar pain. It involves removing a horseshoe shaped strip of skin, eight to 10 mm wide, from the posterior part of the vestibule. The vestibule is part of the vulva between the inner lips, the labia minora, and the ring where the hymen was. Usually, the area of skin excised extends from about 3 o'clock on the left around to 9 o'clock on the right. If symptoms extend further forward, the area removed can be increased towards the opening of the urethra [2].

In some cases, small, isolated areas of skin may be excised from the lower region of the vestibule. Other less common procedures include removing skin close to the back passage, and excising skin from the inner labia (the inner lips of the vagina) [2].

How Long Does the Procedure Take?

The surgery is normally performed under general anaesthesia and takes anywhere from 10 to 40 minutes. Once the affected skin has been removed, the gap between the labia and vagina is closed, and the surgeon stitches the edges together with an absorbable suture. The procedure is usually performed as a day case (meaning the patient does not need to stay overnight), but occasionally the patient will be asked to stay in hospital overnight [2].

How Long is the Recovery Time?

Recovery time is usually rapid, with most discomfort ending within two weeks, though symptoms may remain for up to six weeks. The vulva heals extremely well because of its rich blood supply, so scarring is uncommon. Once healed completely, there should be little to no sign of the surgery at the affected site. Sometimes a vaginal dilator is used post-procedure, and some doctors recommend using a cream such as an emollient or steroid cream. Your surgeon may recommend that you visit a psychosexual counsellor, as PFM spasm can occur with vulvar pain. They may also suggest an appointment with a pain management team, who can carry out a review [2].

Who is a Suitable Candidate?

There are two conditions under the umbrella term of vulvar pain: vulvar vestibulitis (vestibulodynia), and dysesthetic vulvodynia. Surgery is suitable for some women who suffer from vestibulodynia (pain in the vestibule region when touched or provoked). As the Vulval Pain Society notes "This is the classic feature of vestibulodynia, and removal of this tender area of skin will make sense for some women and will be successful. However, overall, vestibulodynia is managed medically, and very few choose to go for surgery. Surgery is rarely carried out for this condition but is effective in well-selected patients" [2].

Women with dysesthetic vulvodynia suffer from more constant pain, and touching the vestibule region may or may not cause additional pain, depending on the individual (studies vary on this point). When women experience constant pain, surgery is less likely to be successful [2].

Are There Any Negative Side Effects?

Adverse effects are rare after vestibulectomy. Most studies report no major complications. Some authors raise the possibility of scar formation and granulation tissue, but these are rare, and the large, published studies suggest a low complication rate [2]. Of course, you should discuss this with your surgeon before undergoing the procedure. It is important to note that, in some cases, surgery may not relieve your pain.

What Does the Research Say?

Reports in medical publications consistently show a high success rate for this procedure, with about 60% complete response (removal of all symptoms) and another 30% partial response (removal of some symptoms). But vestibulectomy shouldn't be thought of as a cure-all. Many factors may contribute to vulvar pain, and it's crucial for surgeons to determine whether or not a person can truly benefit from this surgery before they recommend it.

What Should I Do If My Doctor Suggests Surgery?

Whether you decide to go ahead with surgery or not is a personal choice, but exploring all your non-surgical options first is a good move. The Vulval Pain Society recommends asking your surgeon questions like the following to determine if surgery is right for you:

- Which areas of skin will be removed?
- How long will it take for me to fully recover?
- What is the success rate?
- How many patients have you performed this procedure on?
- What does the outcome audit show?
- What will happen if the surgery fails? [2].

Taking A Closer Look at the Research: Analyzing the Effects of Surgery

One study conducted in 2006 examined the complications and outcomes of surgery for vulvar vestibulitis syndrome. In addition to this, the researchers pinpointed certain patient characteristics that played a role in the outcome [3].

The Method

After reviewing hundreds of medical records, researchers chose 155 women, aged 40 and under, who had undergone a surgical procedure for vulvar vestibulitis one to four years earlier. Via telephone, the researchers spoke to 81% (126 of the 155 subjects) of these women to discuss the resulting complications and outcomes of their surgeries [3].

The Results

Following surgery "93% of the patients could have sexual intercourse compared with 78% before surgery. In 62% of the women, sexual intercourse was painless after surgery. Interestingly, women aged 30 years or younger reported an even higher success rate with sexual intercourse after surgery" [2]. None of the women reported major complications, though the most common side effect was reduced lubrication during sexual arousal, followed by the growth of a Bartholin's cyst (a cyst on one side of the opening of the vagina) [3].

Analysing the Success of Surgery

A similar study from 2008 is entitled "Is Modified Vestibulectomy for Localized Provoked Vulvodynia an Effective Long-Term Treatment? A Follow-Up Study." The researchers of this study re-examined women who had previously met with short-term success for managing localized provoked vulvodynia. Now, they looked at the women's follow-up information to determine the rates of long-term success [4].

The Method

This study was a "retrospective case note review of 110 women with localized provoked vulvodynia and follow-up patient questionnaire. Patients were asked to quantify their pain scores before surgery, at two months after surgery and one year after surgery and score their satisfaction levels" [4].

The Results

During the first year after surgery, the women's average pain scores continued to improve. "The mean score was 9.17 preoperatively, 5.24 at two months after surgery, and 2.48 at one year after surgery" [3]. There was a 7.96 overall mean satisfaction score, and the rates of long-term success mirrored the short-term results [4].

In analysing this study, the National Vulvodynia Association notes that "It is difficult to suggest that surgery is of benefit to all women with vestibulodynia, as this was a well-selected group of women with vulval pain. Did they get better with physical treatment e.g., massage and trainers?" [1].

What's the Takeaway?

"All chronic pain issues are complex, and certainly vulvodynia and vestibulitis represent one of the most challenging chronic pain syndromes" [5].

While, as you can see, many studies show positive results from surgery "most opinion leaders still recommend surgery as the last resort" [5]. And while surgery has been shown to relieve pain in most patients, other treatment methods are still required in many of those cases. More conservative treatments like biofeedback, sexual counselling, and behavioural therapy can also provide relief and improve the sufferer's quality of life.

In a 2006 study by Tommola, P. et al. that selected and reviewed a number of other studies, the authors concluded "Surgery seems effective and safe. Although analysed in 12 studies only, complications are minor, and reversible with no major long-term sequelae" (aftereffect of a disease or injury) [5].

Finally, there is no consensus on the best surgical technique for vulvodynia. There is, however, no doubt that the experience of the surgeon plays a crucial role. Any procedure must encompass all painful areas while avoiding any unnecessary risks [5].

In the end, it's best to discuss the possibility of surgery with your doctor and/or with an experienced surgeon who specializes in this procedure. They can help you decide whether this is the best option for you.

Chapter 23

Relationships and Living with Vulvodynia

"Discussing what vulvodynia is, along with how the pain personally affects you, is crucial, not only for your own well-being, but for your relationships with your partner, family, and close friends" [1].

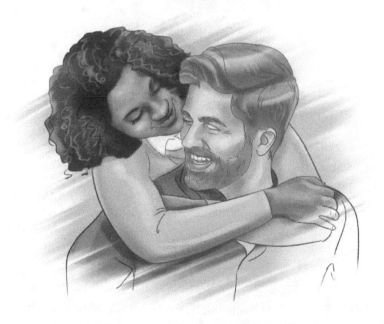

For too long, women suffering from vulvodynia have had to feel that their condition is a taboo subject, and that they must suffer in silence. At long last, this situation is changing. As a Pain Specialist, and as Director of the London Pain Clinic, I am happy to see that my colleagues' efforts in this regard are paying off. This untold suffering of so many women rightfully belongs in the public eye, and should be understood by everyone. That includes your partner.

The National Vulvodynia Association in the US is the world authority on this condition. Their reader-friendly online guide "My Partner Has Vulvodynia – What Do I Need to Know? A Self-Help Guide for Partners" is a must-read for your partner. You can find this resource at www.nva.org/getfile/nva-partner-guide-2016-final-pdf.

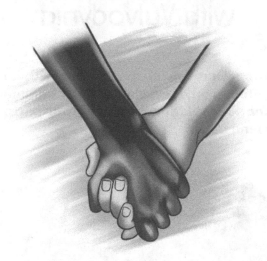

Your Partner Needs to Know What You Are Experiencing

While broaching this subject with your partner is not the easiest thing to do, informing them about your condition can go a long way toward improving your relationship, as well as your own physical and emotional well-being. Being open from the beginning will make it easier to discuss what you are going through with your partner. Hopefully they will be a willing sympathizer and supporter.

For example, if you are going through a flare-up or very stressful phase, your partner may be able to step up and relieve some of your stress load, whether that includes dealing with health insurance companies, paying bills, helping with household chores, or taking care of the children. In fact, your partner could even accompany you to your medical appointments to lend emotional support. Even if not, it's a good idea to share with them your results and treatment options.

This doesn't just have to apply to your partner. You may benefit from having the support and help of other family members and close friends, many of whom probably have no idea what you're going through.

"67% of women with a partner felt comfortable discussing their vulvar pain with them, 39% were comfortable doing the same with family, and 26% with women friends. The more years women had vulvodynia, the less likely they felt comfortable discussing it. Increasing levels of pain were linked to being more comfortable discussing pain with friends" [2].

The above results come from a survey of women with self-reported vulvodynia (which had been clinician-diagnosed). Researchers examined how comfortable the women felt discussing their vulvar pain within different relationships, namely: husband/partner, sister/mother, closest friend, and other female friends. They used different multi-variable models to determine the relationship type and to establish whether vulvar pain characteristics (family history, severity, and time span), played any role in how comfortable the women felt talking about it. The results indicated that "vulvar pain characteristics may determine how comfortable a woman is to discuss her vulvar pain, but it varies by relationship type" [2].

Lifestyle Changes: The Best Strategies for Living with Vulvodynia

It's simply a fact that many women with vulvodynia will need to make lifestyle adjustments. Instead of being discouraged by this, try to see these changes as a positive effort that will help you both mentally and physically. The National Vulvodynia Association offers excellent advice for a broad range of scenarios, all of which are designed to benefit you, your partner, and your family. Let's look at these in more detail.

Different Scenarios

The constancy and severity of your pain will determine what you can and cannot comfortably do. For example, you may not be able to do certain types of work; or you may need help caring for your children or live-in relatives. You may find social engagements and daily chores like shopping difficult. Both you and your partner or family members will need to make adjustments, and it may help to come up with an action plan for when flare-ups happen [1].

Household Responsibilities

You've likely developed a standard pattern for household responsibilities over a number of years. But unless you've also established a plan for when one of you is ill, this pattern is likely to go out the window when you experience chronic vulvodynia symptoms and/or difficult side effects from medication. At this point, you may need your partner to step in and lighten your load.

There are still some positive adjustments you can make, however, that may help you manage household responsibilities. Try standing while doing household chores, if sitting down is too painful. Notice when your pain is at its worst, and if this pain follows a pattern. Keeping a daily pain diary can help both you and your pain specialist, and if you do notice a pattern, you and your partner can plan around it. If your responsibilities become too demanding, you might want to approach a relative or friend for help. If you can afford it, another option might be to pay someone to help you [1].

Parenting

Chronic pain is bound to affect your role as a parent, and your children will probably notice that you are acting differently. It's important to be open with your children as with your partner, though of course, depending on your children's ages, they may not understand all the details of your condition.

If you have young children, explain to them that you are sick or have something wrong with your body, and reassure them that it is not life-threatening, contagious, or anything for them to worry about; it just means you're not quite as lively as usual. You might tell them that you will be trying out different forms of treatment with a specialist, and that you are working on getting better so things can run smoothly again. Let them know that, in the meantime, you are making a few changes, such as getting the family involved in helping, in order to ensure that everything stays on track. Your children may be eager to help out when they learn that you need a little extra assistance.

Since raising children is a full-time job, you may want to enlist the help of a family member or trusted friend. Whether you're a homemaker, a professional working outside the home, or a remote worker, this added help can lift a huge weight from your shoulders. If getting this kind of help isn't possible, consider signing your children up for a day care or after school program [1]. While you may not want to send your children to day care, especially if you're usually at home with them, think of this as simply a temporary arrangement until you can start managing your condition more effectively. Your children may even enjoy the experience, as they will have the opportunity to make new friends.

Career and Job Changes

Although most women suffering from vulvodynia are able to continue working, some are not. If your job involves a lot of sitting, you may want to transition to one where you can stand and/or walk more regularly [1]. If you sit at a computer for hours, talk to your manager about getting a standing desk or making other modifications.

If you are experiencing severe pain for protracted amounts of time, you may be able to take a temporary leave of absence or even resign, and if you are lucky, receive medical insurance benefits [1]. These benefits may come from a private insurance policy or a government disability program. If you are unsure about your entitlement, it's a good idea to investigate as soon as possible. Your insurance representatives and/or HR person may be able to help.

Chapter 24

Sexual Intimacy and Vulvodynia

As many women are all too aware, vulvodynia can make having sex intensely painful. This unbearable degree of pain can lead to a lack of physical contact and, in some cases, even damaging the loving affection that held a couple together and changing the dynamics of a once happy, intimate relationship. It can also be deeply discouraging for young adults who want to experiment with sex and feel like they're missing out on this key life experience.

"Some couples feel mutually resentful of their partner's apparent failure to meet or understand their needs" [1].

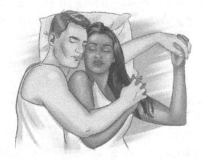

Navigating Relationship Challenges

Vulvodynia sufferers sometimes feel guilty or discouraged when they are no longer able to engage fully in sex with their partner. They may worry that their partner will construe it the wrong way, or that a lack of intimacy will eventually lead to a relationship breakdown.

Unfortunately, those fears are not unfounded. According to one author "a partner, especially a male partner, feels rejected, believing the female partner is exaggerating the pain she feels during sex as a way to brush him off" [1]. On the other hand, if your partner doesn't understand what you're going through, you may find yourself becoming frustrated and resentful.

Of course, sex is not the be-all, end-all of a solid relationship, and not every couple will be affected in this way. But it remains true that "many couples are frustrated by the loss of a way to communicate their love to each other" [1]. In order to preserve your relationship, open communication is key, as we'll discuss in this chapter.

You may also want to read the National Vulvodynia Association's "Overcoming Challenges in Your Intimate Relationship," which you can find at www.nva.org/learnpatient/overcoming-challenges-in-your-intimate-relationship/.

Keeping Your Love Alive

"You may not be able to engage in frequent sexual intercourse, but that doesn't mean your sexual relationship is over. Avoiding all sexual activity can be self-defeating if it leads to a loss of desire in either partner. It is possible to create a satisfying intimate relationship even when you suffer from vulvodynia" [2].

If your vulvodynia pain prevents you from having sexual intercourse for an extended period of time, never fear. There are still plenty of steps you can take to spice up your love life. Oral sex, sensuous massages, whole-body touching, caressing, and kissing are some ideas [3]. If you're in a monogamous relationship, the most important thing is to keep love and affection alive, even if sex is temporarily out of the picture. For example, a kiss and smile when your partner goes out or comes home can go a long way, as can something as simple as holding hands or snuggling on the couch.

"Although vulvodynia is classed as a chronic problem, many women find that their symptoms improve over time, or they find treatments make the condition more

manageable, meaning that sexual activity becomes increasingly pleasurable again" [3].

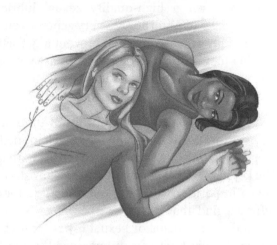

Visiting a Therapist

If you're experiencing relationship challenges, visiting a sex or couples' therapist may be a great way forward [1]. Your therapist may ask how both of you feel about sex, allowing you to separate your feelings about sex from your feelings about each other. If necessary, your therapist may also discuss ways to enjoy sex without the need for penetration, including how to maintain intimacy and/or manage your pain.

If your partner is struggling to understand your vulvodynia, a therapist may be able to help explain things. They might point out to your partner that treatments and disciplines such as Botox, biofeedback therapy, the use of vaginal dilators, and pelvic floor exercises take time to produce results, and that your partner needs to be patient and supportive in the meantime [1]. These types of therapy sessions can help you and your partner grow closer to each other.

Making Penetrative Sex Easier

Penetrative sex is not the only way to enjoy intimacy with your partner. And if penetrative sex is painful for you, your partner should understand that you need to take a break from it for a while. However, if you are looking for ways to make penetrative sex less painful, there are a few things you can try.

First off, get yourself a high-quality sexual lubricant that's recommended for vulvodynia, and apply a very generous amount. This will ensure you are fully aroused and will prevent any friction. Using lidocaine or another topical anaesthetic can help ease your discomfort from penetration [2]. (Note: if your partner is male, he should wear a condom so his penis is not affected by the anaesthetic).

During sex, have your partner spend a lot of time on foreplay. When it comes to sexual positions, some may feel a lot better for you than others, depending on which areas of your vulva are affected by vulvodynia. The key here is to experiment, but also to ask your partner to be gentle, even in positions that are normally fine for you. Most vulvodynia sufferers find that doggy or spooning style (sex in the vagina from behind) with a penis or sexual toy is most comfortable. This makes sense, as this type of sex bypasses the most sensitive regions in your vulva [3].

Several specialists advise women to have regular penetrative sex, but only if they can. Going long periods of time without penetrative sex can generate vaginismus (involuntary spasms of the vaginal wall), making you feel even more tense and uneasy. But the important thing here is to be mindful of your limits. If penetrative sex is too painful, don't do it. Explore other ways to enjoy intimacy until you've found an effective way of managing your condition [3].

Finding What Works

In some cases, it may not be necessary to have a long conversation about vulvodynia in order to communicate to your partner what works and doesn't work. As you experiment with different poses, techniques, and types of sex, pay attention to what brings you pleasure and what brings you pain.

Again, you might try things like oral sex, spooning or doggy style sex, or massages and whole-body touching. You can also use a dilator, as mentioned earlier, to help relax the muscles in your vagina before sex. Listen to your body to find out what excites you and what turns you off or makes you uncomfortable. Then, when you enter a new relationship, you can tell your partner "I like this...." or "I don't like this...." Most people will understand and be considerate even if you don't explain to them that you suffer from vulvar pain.

Whatever you do, don't stigmatize your own experience. Remember that this is a common challenge faced by 16% of women, and that even people who don't suffer from vulvodynia have sexual likes and dislikes. Telling your partner what works and doesn't work for you is a completely normal part of an intimate relationship.

Getting a Conversation Going

In a monogamous relationship, or in a situation where you and your partner are struggling to communicate over this issue, you may benefit from a more serious conversation. Be upfront about your anxieties and worries. Explain the treatments you're taking and what they involve. With that foundation, you can discuss how your intimate relations may need to change. Explain to your partner what gives you pleasure and what brings you pain. Go into as much detail as possible. Tell your partner which vulvovaginal areas and other regions of your body bring pleasure when touched, and which are painful [2]. Below are a few pointers to help you make the most of your conversation.

- **Timing and location are key.** Don't suddenly spring this conversation on your partner. Instead, plan it out in advance. You might even tell your partner that you want to talk to them about this, and together, set a time when the conditions will be right. For example, take time out on a weekend when you are both relaxed, and make sure that you are sitting in a comfortable, private environment.

- **Think through it in advance.** Before your conversation, spend plenty of time thinking about how you really feel. You might even write down some notes. This will help you communicate accurately and cover the important points. You could even do some research beforehand; for example, you might buy a book on oral sex and find a few things you would like to try.

- **Give details.** Go into detail about all the things that bring you sexual fulfilment and pleasure, as well as the things that should (for now at least), be avoided.

- **Respect each other.** Before beginning your conversation, you and your partner should make a mutual promise not to laugh at or embarrass each other. Having a discussion about personal desires and trying out new intimate activities can be sensitive and uncomfortable for both parties, so showing respect and support for each other is crucial.

- **Be a good listener.** Your partner should listen to and respect your concerns. But being a good listener goes both ways. That means considering your partner's point of view and letting them have their say without interrupting. Be patient. Keep in mind that it may take time for your partner to formulate and express their thoughts.

- **Use the 'I' word.** Being a good listener, however, doesn't mean suppressing your own thoughts and feelings. Don't be afraid of using the first person and starting your sentences with "I." "I am really turned on when you...and prefer it to...." "I don't like it when you...as it hurts me." Give your partner positive feedback as well as negative, explaining what works as well as what doesn't.

What Does the Research Say About Your Partner's Response?

Recent studies suggest that "how partners respond can greatly affect the relationship quality of couples affected by vulvodynia. For instance, researchers have found that male partners showing affection and encouraging other kinds of sexual behaviours, leads to better sexual and relationship satisfaction compared to 'solicitous' behaviour (such as suggesting stopping all sexual activity)" [1].

Further, many studies have associated provoked or localised vulvodynia to lowered sexual satisfaction, "but not necessarily to decreased relationship quality, and other research has suggested that even the intensity of the pain women report can be affected by partner responses" [1]. In other words, your relationship can still thrive in the shadow of vulvodynia. Good news indeed!

Chapter 25

Pregnancy and Giving Birth for Vulvodynia Patients

Unfortunately, women with vulvodynia can have a hard time finding medical care for vulvar pain during their pregnancy. In part at least, this may be due to "potential feelings of invalidation when interacting with providers prior to pregnancy; changes to the body experienced during pregnancy; inability to engage in new or medication-based treatments during pregnancy; and the paucity of practitioners specializing in vulvar pain and obstetrics" [2].

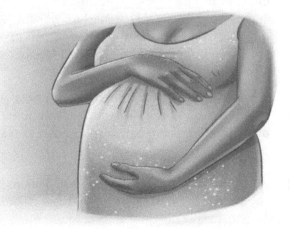

As the BioMed Central Journal notes, even though countless women suffer from vulvodynia, to date, very little has been published regarding "the thoughts, feelings, and experience of vulvodynia patients regarding conception, pregnancy, and delivery. This includes the effect that a hallmark symptom, dyspareunia (painful sex), can have on a couple's physical and emotional ability to conceive" [1]. In this chapter, we'll review some of these very important topics.

Studies on Pregnancy and Vulvodynia

Pregnancy and Pain-Related Anxiety

One study conducted in 2015 interviewed 18 women suffering from vulvar pain. These women were chosen from a potential pregnancy cohort study of women across the UK [1].

The interview uncovered some things that the participants had in common. When describing their response to pain, the women noted that although their pain was volatile in the beginning, "over time, it became more self-controlled, regardless of medical treatment. Once the volatility became more stable and overall severity lessened, many women began planning for pregnancy. Techniques described by women to cope with pain around pregnancy included pain minimization, planning pregnancy-safe treatment, and timing intercourse around ovulation" [1]. Most participants said they felt anxious about how becoming pregnant could affect their pain, yet they all remained hopeful [1].

The women in the study also identified certain strategies. These included "finding a personally acceptable level of pain before planning pregnancy, and a resilience that allowed them to achieve their reproductive goals despite pain and perceived lack of assistance from healthcare providers" [1].

Further research needs to explore the advantages of having more psychosocial support from professionals, husbands, and partners, all of whom could help to improve vulvodynia sufferers' resilience [1].

Pain Catastrophizing

Other research entitled "The vulvodynia patient and pregnancy: a qualitative study on pain catastrophizing and care-seeking behaviors," was carried out in 2014 at the University of Minnesota School of Public Health. This study aimed to learn more about the feelings, thoughts, and experiences of vulvodynia sufferers around delivery, pregnancy, and conception; including the impact of painful sex when trying to conceive [2].

Researchers conducted extensive interviews with 18 women, eight of whom were pregnant, and 10 of whom were in postpartum (post-delivery). Most of these women went through a period of remission while trying to become pregnant "they had reached a point of stability with their symptoms, pain variability, and coping mechanisms" [2].

This study indicates that pain changeability, coping strategies, and the absence of consistently efficient remedies for vulvodynia may affect not only a woman's decision to try for pregnancy, but also her choices regarding delivery method. The participants' sensitivities toward "pain experience during pregnancy and delivery closely fit with a model of pain catastrophizing. Potential interventions to reduce patient anxiety related to the unknown future of their pain should be developed" [2].

Likelihood of Cesarian Sections (C-sections)

Another study undertaken in 2012 examined pregnancy and delivery characteristics of women with and without vulvodynia. Researchers collected data from women aged 18 to 64 who had a history of vulvar pain. 12,047 women were analyzed. Of these, 8,125 (67.4%), filled out a short screening questionnaire which "assessed the history of four types of symptoms that lasted for three or more months, namely itching, burning, knife-like sharp pain, pain on contact (with tampon insertion, intercourse, or pelvic examination)" [3].

When it came to getting pregnant, researchers did not find any significant difference between women with and without vulvodynia. "37% of vulvodynia sufferers who had vaginal delivery, versus 11% of controls, reported pain at two months postpartum. Comparing only women with vulvodynia, women who had intermittent pain versus constant pain were more than twice as likely to have a pregnancy" [3].

However, the study showed that those with vulvodynia were more likely to be given a Cesarean section. In their summary, the researchers found that "women with vulvodynia may be as likely as other women to carry their pregnancy to birth; however, they may experience higher rates of Cesarean section (C-section) delivery" [3].

The Impact of Vulvar Pain on Pregnancy

"Your pain does not mean that you will have increased difficulty birthing the baby" [5].

Some women develop vulvodynia during or just after pregnancy. Others who already have vulvodynia may experience a change in their symptoms, either for better or worse. Of course, every situation is different, and one woman's reaction will not necessarily be the same as another's [4].

"It is possible to have a normal pregnancy and delivery with no ill effects for you and your baby" [5].

Many women worry that vulvodynia will make for a hard pregnancy. While, as discussed above, pregnancy may affect your pain, the Vulval Pain Society points out that "there are no effects of vulvodynia on the outcome of your pregnancy and your baby. This is regarding the growth and overall health of your baby. There is no evidence that women with vulvodynia have a lower normal delivery rate or are more likely to need forceps" [4]. Some women do, however, opt for a Caesarean section when going into labor [4].

Can Pregnancy Impact Vulvar Pain?

Early in your pregnancy, your body produces the hormone oestrogen. Higher levels of oestrogen can actually reduce vulvar pain. But pregnancy can also exacerbate vulvodynia.

Studies show that "women with vulvar pain prior to delivery are more likely to have vulvar pain after delivery" [5]. Similar research suggests that in groups diagnosed with vulvar vestibulitis, "one fifth of women noticed their pain started following delivery. However, it is not clear whether this was true vestibulodynia or pain from other causes (e.g. vaginal stitches or lack of estrogen whilst breast-feeding)" [4].

Pain in the vulvar region has even been reported in women who have given birth by Cesarean section. Those who have given birth to more than one baby appeared to experience varying degrees of pain after delivering different children [4].

The truth is, various issues can cause vulvar pain post-delivery. If you experienced vulvodynia before delivery, there's a possibility that your pain will flare up afterward [4]. Some other causes of post-delivery vulvar pain include:

- Stitches

- Stitches healing too tight (which normally causes painful sex)

- Estrogen deficiency while breast-feeding (which, again, normally causes painful sex)

- Vaginal infections such as thrush [4].

Stitches

If you have a vaginal delivery and experience a tear, you may need stitches. If the stitches are too tight or become infected, they may generate pain in the vulvar region. If this happens to you, book an appointment with your doctor or midwife as soon as possible [4].

Once the vulvar skin has fully healed from being stitched, some women find that having sex is painful. This may be because the stitches left a bridge of skin across the lower section of the vulva. Fortunately, this does not happen very often, but if it does, book an appointment with a gynecologist. They can carry out a minor surgery, called a Fenton's procedure, which releases the skin [4].

Estrogen Deficiency

If you have decided to breastfeed, then because of prolactin (the hormone responsible for breast milk), you are not likely to be ovulating. In that case, your levels of estrogen will be low until your periods resume. If you are low on estrogen, you may experience vaginal dryness and painful sex. If you do, discuss your symptoms with your doctor. You may find water-based lubricants, either with or without a local anesthetic, helpful for the pain [4].

Thrush Infections

In a normal pregnancy, increasing estrogen increases the amount of white discharge from the vagina. It does not produce any irritation or itching. If you do experience itching, you may have a thrush infection in your vagina. For women with vulvodynia, it's important to be aware of thrush infections, as the irritation can worsen your other vulvodynia symptoms. In a thrush infection, you will usually experience itching, followed by soreness and a white discharge like milk curds [4].

If this is the case, visit your doctor. They will take a swab of the discharge and, if you do have vaginal thrush, prescribe an anti-fungal cream or pessary (a device inserted into the vagina). Oral fluconazole and similar medications are not licensed for use during pregnancy and should not be taken. Do not over-treat your condition with anti-fungal creams, as these can cause further irritation and only make your condition worse. Make sure to follow your doctor's advice for all treatments, and don't take a treatment without consulting your doctor first [4].

A Few Tips to Help Minimize Vulvar Pain

As soon as you have given birth to your baby, ask your doctor or midwife to use icepacks to help reduce swelling in the vulvar region. Do not use antiseptics, and be sure to follow good hygiene standards. Local anesthetic sprays and gels applied to the vulva may also help relieve pain in the short term, but they can also cause irritation. You may want to discuss these options with your doctor before delivery [4].

Cesarean Section (C-section)

Naturally, many women worry that a vaginal delivery may worsen their vulvar pain [4]. The Vulval Pain Society notes that "some members... have been so concerned at the thought of a vaginal delivery and its effects on vulvodynia that they have opted for Cesarean section. Having a Cesarean section may possibly (but not totally) prevent a flare-up of your vulvodynia" [4].

If you're considering a C-section, just know that this delivery method includes a six-to-eight-week recovery time. The Vulval Pain Society reports that while "vulvodynia is not a common reason for a Cesarean section, it has been heard of" [4]. If you want to learn more about getting a C-section, talk to your doctor. They can help you weigh the pros and cons of this delivery method.

Talk to Your Clinician about Vulvar Pain

"There are ways to manage the discomfort you may feel with vaginal exams or other parts of the pregnancy, delivery, and recovery" [5].

While midwives, obstetricians, and ultrasound technicians are familiar with pelvic pain issues, you may have to make the first move, as they may not always ask if you have vulvar pain. At your first appointment with one of these professionals, bring up your pain, describe its degree of severity, and explain how it affects you. Since vulvar pain can affect your pelvic exams and delivery anxiety, it's essential to communicate your concerns to your clinician. This in turn can help lessen your anxiety about pregnancy and delivery, and guide the practitioner to give you the type of care you require [5].

Minimize Discomfort During Examinations and Delivery

In order to make your examinations, delivery, and other procedures as comfortable as possible, both physically and emotionally, consider the following tips.

Before delivery, discuss your biggest concerns with your clinician or care team. How will your practitioners handle any complications, and what will they do to reduce risk?

Ask your clinician to be very sensitive of your pain when they carry out your pelvic exam. Ask about the procedure beforehand so you know exactly what to expect. Make sure you are in control of the situation, and that your clinician will stop your pelvic exam if you ask them to. If you prefer, ask if you can insert the vaginal ultrasound transducer yourself.

If you would like to keep some of your own clothes on during examinations and delivery, ask your clinician if this is possible. During the examinations and other procedures, find a comfortable position and tell your clinician that this position is comfortable for you.

Ask your medic to apply maternal directed pushing at the time of delivery.

Ask about what to expect when you are recovering from giving birth [4].

Will Vulvodynia Affect My Baby?

If you have vulvodynia, you don't need to worry that the condition will affect your baby. Research shows that babies born to vulvodynia sufferers "have the same Apgar scores and perinatal mortality as those born to women without pain. Babies of women with vulvar pain also showed no difference in the rate of miscarriages, stillborn, and preterm births. These babies are more likely to be born by Cesarean section, induced labor, or vacuum assisted delivery" [5]. In other words, while vulvodynia may affect your delivery method, it has no effect on your baby.

How Can I Avoid a Perineal Injury?

Most childbearing women are concerned about tears in the perineum, and this is especially true for women with vaginal or vulvar pain. Fortunately, there is no evidence that vulvodynia increases your risk of a perineal tear. On the contrary, studies show that "vaginal delivery is safe even after vestibulectomy and is not associated with more perineal tears" [5]. All the same, if you're concerned about protecting your perineum during childbirth, there are several steps you can take.

1. A Perineal Massage

A perineal massage stretches the muscles and tissues surrounding the vaginal opening. This massage should be carried out during the last few weeks of pregnancy. It may lower your likelihood of needing an episiotomy (a surgical incision made at the opening of the vagina during childbirth to ease a difficult delivery and prevent tissue rupture). And in addition, it may lessen the possibility of getting a large tear, especially for first-time mothers [5].

2. A Warm Compress

While you are in labor, the practitioner assisting your delivery places a warm compress on your perineum and massages your vaginal opening. This hands-on support during delivery of the baby's head minimizes your risk of getting a perineal tear [5].

3. Delivery Position

The position of your body at the time of delivery can affect how easily you give birth. Many mothers "squat to give birth, because it makes the pelvis want to open, and takes advantage of gravity. Side lying or hands and knees provide similar advantages" [4].

4. Maternal Pushing

In maternal pushing, you choose when to push according to your urges. This type of pushing is better for the pelvic floor than the coached method [5].

Can Vulvodynia Medication Affect My Baby?

Pharmaceutical drugs and creams for vulvar pain may pose a risk to your unborn baby. For this reason, if you become pregnant or plan to become pregnant while taking medication for vulvodynia, talk to your doctor as soon as possible. Together, you can discuss which pain-relieving medications and topicals will be safe. It's best to discuss this as soon as you start planning your pregnancy. Safe methods include pelvic physical therapy, acupuncture, and mindful meditation. You can also apply a cool or warm compress in the region where you feel pain [5].

Common painkillers like ibuprofen (associated with Nurofen and Advil) can actually disrupt the fertility cycle, and it's recommended that women avoid using ibuprofen throughout their pregnancy. Most of the time, acetaminophen is considered safe for pregnant women, as are opioids when used in the short term [6]. However, you should still consult your doctor about taking any medication during pregnancy.

Is Pelvic Physical Therapy Safe During and After Pregnancy?

"A physical therapist is a valuable part of your pain management team while trying to conceive, during pregnancy and postpartum" [5].

Subject to a few modifications due to pregnancy, pelvic physical therapy can be safe and very beneficial. If your pregnancy is low risk, internal therapy can offer the same gains. If sexual intercourse is safe for you, "then physical therapy is considered safe. Physical therapy for women with vulvovaginal pain very rarely includes Kegels, instead it is often aimed at releasing tension and regaining muscle length. Physical therapy also helps discomfort during the postpartum period" [5]. Internal treatment recommences at least six weeks after delivery, as soon as the midwife or obstetrician clears you to have intercourse.

The Takeaway

In conclusion, you don't need to worry that vulvodynia will affect your baby, although you should talk to your doctor about any pain medications you are taking as soon as you plan to become pregnant. While you may be more likely to have a C-section, if you end up having a vaginal delivery, you are no more likely to suffer complications than a woman who does not have vulvodynia.

While vulvar pain may make your pregnancy more uncomfortable, there are ways to minimize the pain. One of these is physical therapy, which is beneficial and safe both during and after pregnancy [5]. Talk to your doctor about vulvar pain if you are concerned that it will affect your pregnancy.

Chapter 26

Evidence-Based Medicine

At this point, we've talked about some of the evidence for vulvodynia treatments. But when considering this evidence, it's important to understand the basic principles of evidence-based medicine (EBM). This principle helps us recognize that there are levels of evidence, ranging from the least reliable to the most reliable. The EBM pyramid shows these levels in order.

Level 1:
Systematic
reviews and
meta-analyses

Level 2: Critically
appraised topics

Level 3: Critically appraised
individual articles

Level 4: Randomized controlled trials

Level 5: Cohort studies

Level 6: Case series and case reports

Level 7: Ideas, expert opinions, editorials, anecdotes

At the top of the EBM pyramid is the most reliable evidence: systematic reviews and meta-analyses (statistical analyses of the results of multiple studies). At the bottom is the least reliable evidence: background information and expert opinions. When deciding whether to undertake a certain treatment or intervention for a patient, healthcare professionals must consider the most reliable information. As a patient, you have access to much of the same information online, which you can use to evaluate treatment options.

For example, when it comes to using a medication for vulvodynia treatment, the evidence presented in a systematic review or meta-analysis is much more reliable and accurate than an expert's opinion. This is because the methodology used to create the systematic reviews and meta-analyses is significantly more robust.

For some treatments, for example, surgical intervention, there is a limited number of cases, which means there may not be any high-quality evidence available. In that situation, a healthcare professional should consider the next highest level of evidence when deciding on the efficacy (effectiveness) of a particular treatment option.

Evidence-based medicine allows us to understand the overall effectiveness of a treatment and to see an overview of its main adverse effects. In the EBM pyramid, there are seven levels of evidence. From top to bottom, those levels are as follows:

- **Level 1:** Systematic reviews and meta-analyses
- **Level 2:** Critically appraised topics
- **Level 3:** Critically appraised individual articles
- **Level 4:** Randomized controlled trials
- **Level 5:** Cohort studies
- **Level 6:** Case series and case reports
- **Level 7:** Ideas, expert opinions, editorials, anecdotes

Using PubMed

If you're looking for information on a healthcare-related topic, including vulvodynia and its treatment, we recommend using PubMed.

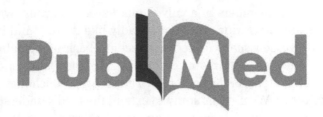

PubMed is the free search engine of the United States National Library of Medicine. It enables you to search more than 30 million resources for biomedical literature, including MEDLINE, life science journals, and online books. Due to rights issues, you may not always be able to view the full text of an article, but you can usually see an abstract and/or summary. If the full text is available, you may find a link to it in the citation.

Healthcare professionals use this site to review the most reliable evidence-based medicine. You can access PubMed at: https://pubmed.ncbi.nlm.nih.gov/.

Evidence-Based Medicine and Online Health Communities (OHCs)

While online health communities (OHCs) can provide helpful support and information, in general, they should not be considered a source of reliable evidence-based medicine.

The following information comes from the 2019 conference paper 'This Girl is on Fire: Sensemaking in an Online Health Community for Vulvodynia," which is available at: https://dl.acm.org/doi/10.1145/3290605.3300359 and https://www.researchgate.net/publication/332747590_This_Girl_is _on_Fire_Sensemaking_in_an_Online_Health_Community_for_V ulvodynia.

"Online health communities (OHCs) allow people living with a shared diagnosis or medical condition to connect with peers for social support and advice. OHCs have been well studied in conditions like diabetes and cancer, but less is known about their role in enigmatic diseases with unknown or complex causal mechanisms.

In this paper, we study one such condition: vulvodynia, a chronic pain syndrome of the vulvar region. Through observations of and interviews with members of a vulvodynia Facebook group, we found that while the interaction types are broadly like those found in other OHCs, the women spent more time seeking basic information and building individualized management plans. They also encounter significant emotional and interpersonal challenges, which they discuss with each other. We use this study to extend the field's understanding of OHCs, and to propose implications for the design of self-tracking tools to support sensemaking in enigmatic conditions" [1].

We'll look at some OHCs for vulvodynia in Chapter 30.

Chapter 27

Ongoing Research Trials for Vulvodynia

Why Is Research Important?

In the last chapter, we discussed using evidence-based medicine to evaluate treatment effectiveness. Medical research is what allows us to do that. Unfortunately, when it comes to vulvodynia treatments, that research still has a long way to go. The following information comes from the National Vulvodynia Association (NVA) website:

"Health care providers who treat vulvodynia do not have evidence-based guidelines to help them select the most appropriate treatment for each patient. Although there are 30 possible treatments to relieve symptoms, there is little, if any, controlled research on most of them. Thus, the burden is on the patient to determine the efficacy of each treatment, a trial and error process that often takes several years.

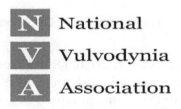

N National

V Vulvodynia

A Association

Although clinical research is lacking, the NVA has awarded over 50 grants to study the potential causes of vulvodynia. Once they establish the cause(s), researchers will understand what treatment(s) need to be developed. To date, the NVA has spent one million dollars on grants awarded from the NVA Medical Research Fund and the Career Development Award to help researchers collect pilot data, so they can subsequently obtain larger grants from major institutions, such as the National Institutes of Health. Some of our grant recipients have been successful in obtaining multimillion-dollar grants from the National Institutes of Health, the Canadian Institutes of Health Research and other institutions.

To increase awareness of research pertaining to vulvodynia and other vulvar pain conditions, the NVA maintains a reference list of all medical research published on chronic vulvar pain disorders since 1965 and provides a biannual update on recently published studies" [1].

Can I Participate in a Vulvodynia Study?

The truth is, we need high-quality clinical trials to examine the effectiveness of different therapeutic approaches for vulvodynia; and we need them now. Currently, approximately 82 ongoing research trials in facilities and universities worldwide are seeking effective treatments for vulvodynia.

You may be able to participate in some of these studies, depending on various criteria, including your location. You can find a list of worldwide trials, and see which trials you may be able to participate in, in the NIH (National Institutes of Health) 'Clinical Trials' section of the U.S. National Library of Medicine website. The web address for this site can be found at the end of this chapter.

Some Clinical Terms

To help you understand what these trials consist of, let's briefly review some terms.

Randomized Controlled Trial (RCT): In a randomized controlled trial, participants get randomly assigned to one of two groups, the experimental group or the control group.

Experimental Group: This is the group that receives the treatment or intervention being tested.

Control Group: This group receives a different treatment, such as a placebo, sham, or conventional treatment. The results of the experimental group are then measured against the results of this group.

Placebo/sham: A placebo is a substance that has no effect. For a sham treatment, the clinician goes through the motions of administering the treatment without actually doing so.

Double-blind: In a double-blind study, neither the study's participants nor the researchers know who is receiving which treatment. This is done to prevent bias.

An Overview of Some Current Trials

Many of these trials are due to end in 2022 or 2023. New trials which extend after these years are automatically listed on the NIH Clinical Trials list, as and when they begin.

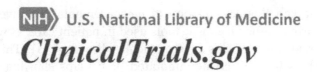

NIH⟩ U.S. National Library of Medicine
ClinicalTrials.gov

Low-Level Laser Therapy for Reducing PVD (provoked vestibulodynia)

"Low Level Laser Therapy is a therapeutic modality involving irradiation of injured or diseased tissue with a combination of red and infrared light. The process is thought to initiate a series of physiological reactions within the cells exposed to light at these wavelengths, leading to the restoration of normal cell structure and function. The investigators hypothesise that this will reduce pain and improve sexual function among women with PVD" [1].

This double-blind randomized controlled trial seeks to determine whether or not

BioFlex™ low-level laser therapy (LLLT) can help relieve PVD. This will involve a partly standardised protocol in regard to: the subjects' physiological responses to pressure on the vulvar vestibule; and self-reported sexual functioning and pain; as well as phasic and tonic activation of the pelvic floor muscles and cerebral cortex excitability to the pelvic floor muscles in PVD patients (with/without co-occurring VAG (vaginismus), when likened to the same schedule of treatment in which sham LLLT is administered [1].

Vulvovaginal Laser Therapy

The goal of this randomized double blinded sham-controlled clinical study is to determine the safety profile, acceptance, and efficacy of vulvovaginal laser therapy in vulvodynia patients. The main study hypothesis is that "laser therapy will be more effective than sham laser therapy in vulvar pain reduction measured by Q-tip test and tampon test." The secondary hypothesis is that "laser therapy, in comparison to sham laser therapy, will lead to more improvement of sexual health and HrQoL [health-related quality of life] will have similar rates of side effects" [1].

Diagnostic Testing: Thermographic Imaging and Mechanical Pain Assessment

"Through this combination of measurements, the investigators plan to expand the diagnostic tools used in patient care, as well as on the classification of this heterogeneous disorder" [1]. This study's researchers hope to create annotated pain maps showing both the regions and sizes of areas that are sensitive to mechanical stimulus. To achieve this, they will use a combination of clinical input, photographs, and infrared images, and will also consider participants' comorbidities (other existing conditions). Infrared imaging will gauge increased skin temperature and areas of inflammation. Using a cotton swab, researchers will produce thermographic images according to a participant's response to mechanical stimulation, and will set pain maps over these thermographic images [1].

Acupuncture for the Treatment of Vulvodynia

This study will evaluate the effectiveness of acupuncture for vulvodynia treatment, particularly regarding painful intercourse and generalised vulvar pain. Researchers will analyse how long the acupuncture's positive effects last. Participants who experience reduced pain after initial treatment will be monitored for pain once per week for up to 12 weeks [1].

The Effect of Thoracic Spine Manipulation on Vestibule Pain

The idea behind this study is to see how thoracic spine manipulation impacts vestibule pain, as observed by sensory testing (Q-tip and pressure algometry) in a group of patients suffering from PVD. The researchers hope to compare the immediate impact of manipulation and sham manipulation with sensory testing of the vestibule or external vulva [1].

Somatocognitive Therapy for Treating PVD

Somatocognitive therapy (SCT) is an aspect of multi-modal physiotherapy aimed at alleviating persistent musculoskeletal pain. In the past, this method was used to treat patients with long-term pelvic pain. This randomized clinical trial analyses the effectiveness of somatocognitive therapy compared to general treatment for PVD [1].

The test subjects will be "assessed at baseline, after 6 months and 12 months. The main outcome will be changes in the female sexual function index scored at 12 months follow up. Secondary outcomes include pain intensity (assessed by a tampon test), as well as questionnaires recording different aspects of emotional and cognitive function" [1].

Lipofilling For the Treatment of Vestibulodynia

In this controlled intervention study, one group will receive vestibulectomy (the 'gold standard' therapy), while the other receives vestibular lipofilling. Researchers will try to determine whether lipofilling with its adipose-derived stem cells might be a less invasive but "equally or more effective therapeutic option for women with vestibulodynia than vestibulectomy" [1]. The researchers are cautiously optimistic, since adipose tissue-derived stem cells have proven effective for reducing inflammation in various forms of neuropathic pain disorder (these include mastectomy pain syndrome and pudendal neuralgia) [1].

Examining the Mutual Link Between Psychosocial Traits and the Progression of Vestibulodynia

This research will analyse how behavioural and emotional responses, cognitive factors, and personality characteristics of participants with localised PVD influence sexual functioning, emotional health, pelvic floor rehabilitation, provoked pain levels, adherence to therapeutic interventions, and the natural history of the syndrome [1].

NIH Clinical Trials Website

You can search for ongoing trials at:

- https://clinicaltrials.gov/

Information on how to use the site is found here:

- https://www.nih.gov/health-information/nih-clinical-research-trials-you/finding-clinical-trial

Chapter 28

Patient Stories

Every woman who has battled vulvodynia has her own story to share. Hearing about other people's experiences can help you realize that you're not alone in this struggle. Vulvodynia is a common condition. In this chapter, we share the stories of women treated at the London Pain Clinic in Harley Street, UK. These women have our tremendous gratitude for their willingness to describe their personal journeys honestly and openly.

The National Vulvodynia Association (NVD), a non-profit organization, has a very inspiring section on their website for patient stories, entitled "Real Women. Real Pain. Real Hope." We share one of those stories here as well.

It Takes Someone Who Has Suffered to Understand

If you know someone who suffers from vulvodynia and are trying to gain a better understanding of this condition, this chapter can help you as well. "Look into the eyes of a woman with vulvodynia and you'll see your mother, your daughter, your sister, your friend. Every day, millions of women of all ages and races worldwide are dealing with this mysterious condition that causes chronic vulvar pain. Sadly, to date, there is no definitive cure" [1]. At the same time, however, "Look closer into the eyes of a woman with vulvodynia and you'll also see the shining rays of hope. Hope that there will one day be a cure that will end her suffering and allow her to resume a normal life again, pain free" [1].

Real Stories from Women Who Chose to Fight Back

Courage and positivity, plus a whole lot of tenacity, are essential for fighting vulvodynia. Let's take an up-close and personal look at some of the inspiring women who chose to share their stories. These women's names have been changed to protect their identities.

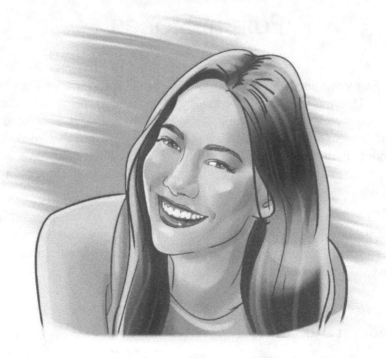

Maria's Story

I developed the first symptoms of vulvodynia when I was 16-17, and my experience with vulvodynia has been defined by facing it as a young person with very little idea of what it was.

I am unsure what may have triggered the onset—I had only recently become sexually active, using the utmost precaution, and, although I once took antibiotics for cystitis, I am not sure if the first onset of pain was related to this infection.

Worried about having an STI (which to a 16-17-year-old seemed like the end of the world) I did a screen through my GP (general practitioner). I am sure that anyone with vulvodynia will understand the incredible pain of a routine STI swab—the thought of that speculum still makes me shudder. The STI screen came back clean, which my young self interpreted as perhaps, the pain was in my head, or at least a normal part of intercourse to be accepted.

The pain began gradually and increased during intercourse which, I am now ashamed to say, I did not (out of embarrassment) disclose to my partner, but instead attempted to mask that I was in pain.

This pain which was increasing consistently was an embarrassment I carried silently, ending, and not allowing myself to enter any relationships for the fear that I would be discovered to be broken or unclean. My 17-year-old self genuinely believed this meant I would always be alone, and because I kept it a secret, no one could have told me otherwise.

Ashamed to admit to my parents that I needed help with such a delicate subject, and with my GP insisting that as I did not have any issues with my sexual health, I finally saved up some money to attend a private appointment. I was turned away from the clinic due to being a month away from being eighteen and told that I could only attend with a parent or guardian.

Finally gathering the courage to speak to my parents, I was given money to attend an appointment with a gynecologist at London Medical, and was given the same STI swab. After another traumatizing experience with a speculum (the most suitable comparison I can think of is intercourse with a Japanese knife), my tests came back clear. My doctor suggested that although the swab tested negative for herpes, he believed that to be the case. I was prescribed acyclovir, which I began taking.

Of course, the symptoms persisted, as did my bewilderment at where this mysterious herpes could have come from. After years of obsessive googling and finding some scarce mentions of a condition called vulvodynia, I tentatively asked whether my symptoms could be that. The doctor I was seeing at London Medical told me the condition was rare and unlikely to be the case.

Frustrated with gynecologists, I went to a dermatologist, thinking that perhaps it was a dermatological issue. It was in this examination where I was told that my symptoms and physical signs showed a clear picture of vulvodynia. When I asked what there was to be done, the doctor's words were a clear "nothing." I was told that I was "still young," that "sometimes just knowing what it is makes people feel better," and that "maybe it will go away." At that stage, I remember very vividly leaving the clinic and sitting down on the curb of a busy street in Chelsea, in the middle of the day, to cry my eyes out. Through all this turmoil, I must note, my mental health has declined to a point where somehow this episode was not even rock bottom.

If there is one thing I am trying to say with this patient story, it is that the stigmatization and lack of awareness about conditions such as vulvodynia (both in general, and most strikingly, amongst medical professionals) can be incredibly damaging to a young person.

As I grew older, I was able to grow accustomed to the diagnosis, although I still suffer with the use of sanitary products and am still not able to wear some clothing items and completely gave up attempting certain types of intercourse. Despite what I had previously thought, I was finally able to allow myself to date (albeit still dreading the inevitable conversation where I had to explain vulvodynia), to discover that most people are more compassionate than I believed them to be.

I have only recently restarted my attempts to find treatment for my vulvodynia, which was due to having finally received a diagnosis and treatment for another health issue which I was previously told could not be helped. This inspired me to search for treatments for vulvodynia, which is how I found Dr. Jenner at the London Pain Clinic.

Speaking to Dr. Jenner has given me a lot of hope, as did him laughing out loud about the claim that there was nothing I could do. I am hopeful that any one of the very many treatments available to me will work, and I am confident that one of them will.

Although I am still hopeful that one day, I will be able to consider my vulvodynia a mere annoyance of the past, being able to discuss it freely with doctors like Dr. Jenner who are informed and understanding of the condition has lifted a huge weight off my shoulders. I can only hope that an increased awareness and decreased stigma of such conditions will be available for young people as I wish it had been for me.

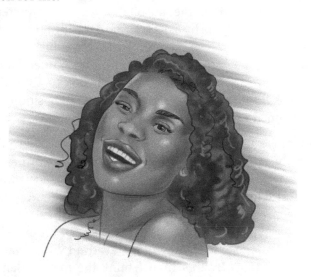

Karen's Story

I first started having problems with vulval pain in around 2013 after a nasty bout of reoccurring thrush. My initial symptoms were a burning and stinging sensation on the entrance to the vagina. It was not something I had suffered with before so the first thing I did was visit my local sexual health clinic for a full check up to make sure everything was okay. After an all clear result I booked to see my doctor (I was at university at the time). It is embarrassing for most people to discuss their genitals in general so I was nervous about speaking to the doctor and the first appointment I had was horrible. The doctor wouldn't believe me when I'd said I had the all clear from the GUM clinic. She made me feel really small and was insistent that I do another chlamydia test even though I'd told her I had recently had a negative test result. I refused to do another test after explaining to her that even a cotton swab up there was causing me severe pain and I wasn't willing to do another so soon after having the all clear. I think the doctor had judged me based on my age, looks and the fact I was at university. After leaving the doctors in tears I went back to my partner and we decided we would just keep trying to have sex and hope that my symptoms would die down soon.

On realising the symptoms were only getting worse I decided to book to see a different doctor to try and get to the bottom of the problem. I was then referred to see a gynecologist at a nearby hospital. After my appointment at the hospital I felt much better, I was diagnosed with vulvodynia by a doctor who described the burning and stinging sensation was caused by my muscles spasming and tightening around anything that entered my vagina. His recommendations were to relax during penetration and realise that eventually my muscles would relax as they couldn't stay in the contracted position "forever". He recommended I was seen again in six months time.

Six months later and I was still having problems and feeling quite upset with the situation. During my follow up appointment I saw a different doctor who confirmed that the original diagnosis was correct and that all still looked healthy with my vagina. When I mentioned I was still having pain the doctor prescribed lidocaine gel and suggested I put it in my vaginal entrance twenty minutes prior to sex to see if that would help. Feeling again slightly more positive I went away with the lidocaine to try that. By this time I think the mental damage had already been done and the lidocaine didn't really help because I didn't like the thought of having to "plan" sex with a twenty minute warning.

After this I just turned off any emotions or needs to sex and would avoid it. I have been with my partner since the start of my problems so I think someone should give him a medal. A few years went by of me shrugging it off and feeling embarrassed at any social event where the discussion of sex and intimacy would come up. I would either talk about something from years before or just try to change the subject, something no one should have to do (especially in your twenties)!

I went back to my GP in 2018 and discussed my problems. It is worth adding that for every doctor I have seen, I have had to describe what vulvodynia is as they don't seem to know. I think this shows how unspoken about vulval pain is in general. She checked my vagina and confirmed all looked healthy and we discussed options. We agreed that she would refer me for some psychosexual therapy to see how that would help. This was in December 2018 and knowing the strain on the NHS I didn't think anything of it when I hadn't received my invitation to a first appointment 6 months later. I called my GP surgery to ask about the referral and they said she had referred me and to wait. To this date I never received an appointment so sadly I'm not confident it was ever made.

In July 2019 after suffering with acne for years I went to see my local private GP in London after making the most of private healthcare through my work insurance. In this appointment I also discussed how both my acne and vulval pain were making me feel very low. The Doctor immediately referred me to a dermatologist for my acne (I can now say I've been acne free for a year) and to a specialist for my vulval pain. After my initial appointment with the specialist, I was prescribed a steroid cream to apply on the area twice a day and lidocaine to use every night before bed. I had a follow up with the specialist a few months later and after no real change in my pain, she referred me to a pain specialist.

Unfortunately my insurance would only cover a small amount of the pain specialists fee and I was unable to pay the difference especially when not knowing the treatment I would need and this additional cost. After seeing me in floods of tears (which I think was my pure disappointment), my partner googled vulvodynia pain and came across the London Pain Clinic. After reading the testimonials on the website I contacted my insurance who confirmed they would cover the cost of an initial consultation with Dr Jenner. After my initial appointment with Dr Jenner I felt a small wave of relief. Although our appointment had to be via phone call (due to Covid-19) Dr Jenner came across as calm and reassured me that there were lots of different treatment options for me. He explained that one size doesn't fit all in the treatment of vulval pain but he wrote me a list of options. After this initial appointment we confirmed I would start on pain relief tablets (pregabalin) and also a specially made ointment to use internally twice a day (gabapentin 6%).

One month on I had a follow up consultation with Dr Jenner and he then referred me to a pelvic physiotherapist. I wasn't sure what to expect from my first appointment with the physio but after my first appointment with her I cried with relief and thought, she is going to be able to help me. I have now been seeing the physio for around six months and the change has been huge. She firstly recommended some exercises based on strengthening up my glute muscles and ensuring I wasn't putting any extra strain on my pelvic floor (something I've only thought you talk about after you have children). She then started teaching me how to contract and release using my pelvic floor which seems simple but it has taken a lot of practice. After this she recommended the use of dilators which have made a huge difference to my life so far. Over the last few months I have gone from only just about being able to put in the smallest dilator (around the size of a small tampon) to being able to insert the largest one. Since the treatment started I have started using tampons for my period which I was unable to use before and have managed to have sex twice - realise this doesn't sound like a lot but this was a huge step in the right direction. For someone who has suffered with this for so long, it feels amazing to be where I am right now with my treatment and I feel like the future is bright. I also feel confident that if my current treatment doesn't quite do the trick that there are many avenues to explore with the help of Dr Jenner and the London Pain Clinic.

Vulval pain has life changing consequences, not being able to have sex and losing the relationship with your vagina makes you feel really low. It also makes planning for the future difficult. The fact I have had to go through a private clinic to get the treatment I need after years of trying through the NHS shows how unheard of and unspoken about vulval pain is. I think this is something which has to change moving forward as not everyone has the privileged option of private medical insurance. If I could give any advice to myself all those years ago or to someone suffering now it would be to be more forward and push for what you think you need. Don't be embarrassed and acknowledge that this is a pain like any other and it needs treatment.

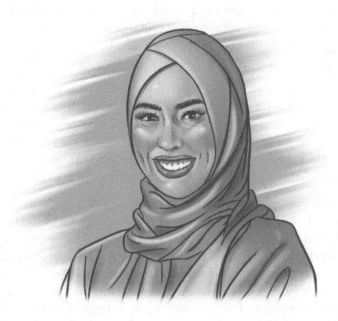

Angela's Story

"My problems began in the summer of 2019 when I got a vaginal infection. I saw various consultants at that stage who struggled to find the cause of my problem. It was extremely uncomfortable: itching, prickling, and a constant pain, as well as a nasty discharge. Once the infection cleared finally with antibiotics, the itching, prickling, and pain in my vulva did not improve at all. If anything, it all became worse.

I saw various gynecologists over several months who told me that there was nothing wrong with me. I was swabbed for everything under the sun and everything came back clear. By this time, I was really struggling not only physically but mentally. I felt that, if I did not get some relief from this problem, I could not really face carrying on with my life. Everything suffered: work, my home life, and my friends. I became quite isolated and depressed and cried every day.

I had several counselling sessions at this time. Fortunately, my work provided an employee helpline which funded 10 sessions. The counselor made me see that I needed to seek alternative opinions and that I was not at the end of the road. It really made me feel less despondent about my life and I would urge anyone suffering with this awful problem to seek appropriate mental health support.

Eventually, I saw a new gynecologist who said that he thought I had vulvodynia. I had never heard of this condition, but it certainly matched my symptoms. He referred me to Dr. Chris Jenner at the London Pain Clinic who had experience treating this condition. He made me feel better when he said he saw four women a week with this problem and he understood the impact on my physical and mental health. He gave me hope that there were options to help me, but explained that it could be trial and error with several medications.

I have been with Dr. Jenner now for probably eight months and during that time, we have tried several combinations of medications. Now, I think I am 80% better—which is amazing. I can go for a full day without symptoms, though I still have bad days. Dr. Jenner tweaks my medications to help offset the side effects (tiredness, mostly) and has frankly saved me. I do not really like shoveling so many tablets into my body every day, but medications are there for a reason and sometimes, we all need help.

Do not suffer in silence with this illness. It is not in your mind; you just need to find the right doctor to help you. My experience is that this is a little-known and little-understood condition, and you need to find a pain expert who knows what they are talking about. Hope this account helps others avoid going through the same misery as I have for the last year or so.

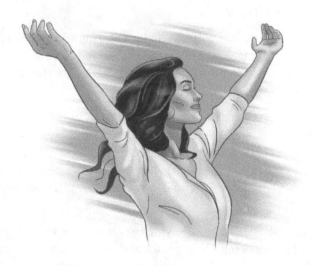

Sandra's Story

Sandra's symptoms first surfaced after an egg collection procedure about 18 months ago. She describes them as being "knife-like pains that made intercourse really painful; as well as a constant sensation of dryness" [2].

Her life was negativity affected as she completely lost her libido. This lack of sex drive brought about by a combination of mental and physical factors naturally caused her distress.

She first sought help around six months ago, a year after she fist experienced vulvodynia symptoms. Her gynecologist was unable to help her, but referred her to other doctors, namely "a vaginal pain specialist, a women's physiotherapist, and then Dr. Jenner" a pain specialist at the London Pain Clinic [2].

Sandra said that she first had physiotherapy, then tried pulsed radio frequency to the pudendal nerves, and that the latter worked for her. Commenting on how her symptoms feel now, she said "I feel much less pain now, things are almost back to normal" [2]. Excellent news indeed!

Sandra advises: "for those who want almost immediate results, pulsed radio frequency [is a] low risk procedure with no need for medication. Pulsed radio frequency [could be] the right treatment for you. It really helped remove my pain within a couple of weeks" [2].

Elizabeth's Story

"I felt a strange feeling like a paper cut around my vulva. Then a nerve started pinging, and I began to feel sore. It was also painful to sit down. I went to the doctor, who told me it was thrush, and so I went on a course of antibiotics [2].

My condition never improved, so I kept going back and forth to the doctors who examined me and said everything was fine. [All they did was] prescribe some cortisol cream. On my fourth visit, I demanded to see my designated doctor, who prescribed me a low dose of amitriptyline. On my fifth visit, my doctor said I needed to see a gynecologist [2].

By this time, it felt like someone was sticking a red-hot poker up inside me; I was in excruciating pain and experienced a great deal of tingling. It seemed like I had a golf ball stuck inside me, and I had a dragging feeling along with muscle spasms. I could not work, so I went on sick leave. I kept crying, and my husband did not know what to do. I had to lie on my side (the one that wasn't affected), just to eat and rest, and spent most of the day walking around the house in pain! [2].

I saw a gynecologist who said I had to have a vulva biopsy, as the condition could be Lichen sclerosis [a skin condition which produces itchy white patches on the genitals/other parts of the body]. About three weeks later when I had this done, I was in even more pain. To relieve the latter, the gynecologist prescribed codeine, but this gave me very bad constipation [2].

I was now very depressed and suicidal. When I had my follow-up appointment, I was given all clear for Lichen sclerosis, but was diagnosed with vulvodynia. Several different medications and a nerve block were suggested. After six months of constant severe pain, I was so pleased to be having treatment [2].

I had a nerve block procedure, which was undertaken by the NHS (National Health Service in the UK). During the weeks I waited for the nerve block, I was at my worst, and just wanted to end my life" [2].

But instead of the nerve block treatment turning things round, to Elizabeth's dismay, the procedure did not work. "I was still in excruciating pain and couldn't sit" [2].

To help alleviate the pain, Elizabeth ordered and tried out several orthopedic cushions. In addition to this, she started using a TENS machine to see if it could help her when she was sitting down, but she says, "I was still in pain. At this stage, and for several weeks, I was in such pain that I was prescribed oramorph (liquid morphine), which I started to take daily. This helped me a little" [2].

"Not long after this, I had another follow-up meeting with the consultant, and was told that there was nothing more that could be done. I was subsequently referred to a vulva clinic, where I was told that I could have another nerve block if I wanted to go through the procedure again [2].

Because I was so fed up and annoyed, I had a look around at what could be done privately, and eventually went to a private pain clinic in Hampshire, UK. The pain clinic prescribed me Gabapentin (to be taken along with amitriptyline, which I was already on). I also had an MRI scan (which the NHS never offered at any stage); but when the results came back, no problems were detected. I was then referred to a spinal surgeon, who performed an epidural procedure to 'wash through' the lower spine with a steroid [2].

The epidural didn't work, so I was back to square one. The spinal surgeon contacted the vulva clinic consultant and suggested that a further nerve block procedure should be carried out. When I came round from the anesthetic, and was back on the ward, I was told yet again that they could not do any more, and did not even want to see me for a follow-up. They told me to go down the physio route and I would need to look further afield myself [2].

The nerve block didn't work, so my pain continued, as did the tingling sensation; and I still couldn't sit. I was forced to return to work, because I was told that I would lose my job if my absence continued. While at work, I used the TENS machine as a means of pain relief almost all the time. But even with this, and sitting on a cushion, I was still in pain. I did not want to go out anywhere, and life was miserable. What I was going through, and the way it affected me, was making my husband annoyed with me, and things were getting to a point that I worried he would leave me [2].

After having conducted numerous internet searches, I finally came across the White Hart Clinic in London, UK, which offered to help me; and I started physiotherapy. At last, I had found someone who understood the condition and listened to me" [2]. To get to this stage, Elizabeth's quest to heal her vulvodynia, had taken well over a year.

She notes "the physiotherapist at the White Hart Clinic not only undertook physiotherapy, but also showed me a number of exercises that would help. I am still going to the White Hart Clinic every few months and am doing physio exercises every other day. The clinic also advised meditation, which I continue to do [2].

This has helped me tremendously, but the pain still remained, and so I continued looking for further help. Then, I came across the London Pain Clinic via the internet and arranged to see Dr. Jenner. At last, I had found a consultant who listened and understood. My medication was changed to different doses to see what would work best, and I felt more confident going there [2].

One of the options I discussed with Dr. Jenner was Ultrasound Guided Pulsed Radio frequency. I underwent the procedure. Following the treatment, I initially felt uncomfortable for a few weeks, but then things started to improve, and gradually I felt so much better [2].

With the help of the physiotherapist at the White Hart Clinic, and the treatment at the London Pain Clinic, my life is now so much better. The pain and tingling have considerably improved, and I can now sit without a cushion for a small amount of time [2].

I am not working now, so my stress levels have gone down, which has also helped. I am about 80% well now and can look forward to leading a more normal life. I still get the odd days where I feel uncomfortable, and still cannot sit for long periods of time, but I do have more good days than bad [2].

I would advise other sufferers to seek help as soon as possible, and to get a good physiotherapist who understands vulvar pain. Do research on the internet, and do not give up. I know this is difficult, but there is help there. I was lucky enough to go privately to the London Pain Clinic, and I would thoroughly recommend them" [2].

Deborah's Story

"I had vulvodynia in the beginning of 2017, but looking back, there were moments when I thought it was thrush, so I had treatment and thought that the symptoms would pass. Later in the year, the symptoms in my urethra, vagina, and part of my perineum (the region between the anus and vulva), became worse, and I went to see a specialist [2].

It killed me. I've stopped working; I'm depressed; I've put on weight; I'm swollen; I'm not the person I used to be. I cannot remember the last time I really laughed… how sad. How is it that doctors do not know enough about vulvodynia? I am pain free, but that is due to all the meds. I don't feel I'm better; I will feel better once I can lower the meds [2].

Some [consultants] are happy to give you pills, and others are trying to get you off the pills, regardless of the fact that I keep telling them that in the past, when I lowered my meds, the pain returned [2].

If only the first doctor who had diagnosed vulvodynia had introduced me to nortriptyline at an early stage, I would not be on such a high dose. If only I had seen Dr. Jenner sooner [2].

Now, I don't feel pain, apart from the time it stops working, and you have to up the dosage again; or when I am trying to lower it [2].

Do your own research, and don't take no for an answer if the doctor tells you it's nothing and it's all in your head. See a couple of specialists to get an idea of which direction you need to go in; and say some prayers. Inform your partner and get them to understand so you have a support system. You may find that some relatives do not believe you, because this headache is invisible, and you can get good days as well as bad [2].

Most importantly, find someone who is also going through this, and chat to them. You need to talk to an existing patient so you can get all the information that has not been written down. Unfortunately, from all the specialists that I have seen, none of them have this service, which is a shame, as it could help so much. Women are afraid to talk because it's in an intimate area [2].

I am looking to write a blog about this headache between my legs, but if there was a service that enables patients to talk to someone who has it or has had it; or maybe a service which could collaborate with a vulvodynia specialist, such as Dr. Jenner, who could provide advice, it could be very beneficial" [2].

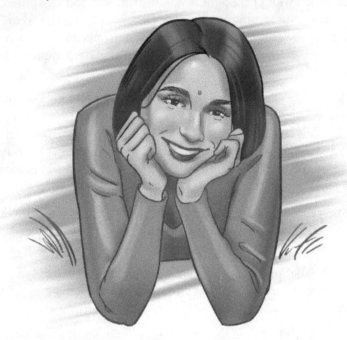

Barbara's Story

"I think I was about 19 years old and had a nasty case of cystitis. Around this time, I also began to get thrush after being more sexually active. After repeated infections, I noticed that the pain would continue long after the antibiotics had finished. I would sometimes also experience pain during and after sex, which would last anything between a few hours to a few days/weeks. My two worst flare ups lasted around two years each. Not pleasant!

[Symptoms included] extreme soreness and burning pain mainly around the clitoral area. I once heard someone describe it as a "Chinese burn x 1000, and this is exactly how it feels. I have cystitis-like symptoms, along with diarrhea and bowel pain. Often, I would wake up needing to pee at four AM and would be unable to get back to sleep, so I would become very tired. The thrush also comes and goes, but I have avoided sugar and yeast for many years now, and this seems to help [2].

In later years, I have experienced vaginal soreness during and after sex, which luckily, has always gone away. The clitoral pain lingers, however. It may also be worth mentioning that I had no symptoms throughout any of my three pregnancies, or while I was breastfeeding. I have wondered whether this was because I had something else to think about that was positive. I am sure that psychology and stress have a massive bearing on this condition [2].

It has definitely affected my sex life, and my marriage as a result. I have lost my sex drive completely, and associate sex with pain, so I am reluctant to try. I am unable to go into very cold or very hot water (it sets the pain off), so I do not swim any more. I also avoid horse riding and cycling. I used to jog, but have stopped that also, as it would sometimes set off the pain. I have had feelings of depression, loneliness, frustration, anger. I look at other people and feel resentment that they are healthy and I am not.

Whenever I have an episode of vulvodynia, I feel quite traumatized, and it brings back many sad, awful, desperate feelings. I am quite a strong person, but whenever this condition rears its ugly head, I totally fall apart! I can say it has ruined my life over the years, and to this day, I am unable to have a healthy sex life/intimate relationship with my husband. The way I feel now is that I never want to have sex again, and I am only 47 years [old]. I have no idea how to get over this! [2].

Over the years I have seen dozens of doctors and specialists, and it has only been in the last 12 months that I have heard the terms vulvodynia and clitorodynia. I feel sad, as that is a lot of wasted time on misdiagnosis! [2].

This is a list of the treatments and investigations I've tried:

- Amitriptyline
- Acupuncture
- Reiki
- Antibiotics & thrush treatments
- Cystoscopy investigations
- Colonoscopy investigations [2]

[Barbara notes that regarding the cystoscopy investigations, the procedures did not work and gave her cystitis [2].]

Reiki may have helped, but I'm not 100% sure. Maybe the pain was passing, anyway. I am currently on Citalopram (30mg per day), and that has worked very well. I still have the odd moment of discomfort, but so far so good. I am going to stay on the treatment for the foreseeable future [2].

I'm feeling much happier and more positive. I still do not feel ready to have sex, so need to deal with those issues and talk it through with my husband. This has been difficult, and to be honest, I keep putting it off. He is aware of my illness but doesn't really understand the full impact it continues to have on my life and emotions [2].

Try to go for a pee often; sometimes holding it in can cause soreness. Avoid hot and cold water, clitoral stimulation during sex, bike riding, and horse riding. Try and avoid getting things like thrush and UTIs, as they set off a chain reaction. Try and stay positive. When I am busier, the pain improves. Do not sit around and worry about it if you can. Stay active and try to stay happy. I know it's very hard!" [2].

Mary's Story

"I remember lying on the bathroom floor thinking: what's wrong with me? I did not have a way to talk to anyone about it. And so, I did not. It was my secret, private pain" [1].

While it's not unusual to hear people talk about physical therapy, Mary points out, when it comes to pelvic floor physical therapy, that's a whole different ball game. "It involves having your insides massaged through your most intimate opening" [1]. It is needed because "your vagina hurts. It has always hurt" [1].

Her vagina has never felt sensual or sexy, and she has never had any pleasurable sensations connected to her intimate region which she succinctly describes as throbbing, stabbing, and burning [1]. Mary, who is 33 years old, remarks "I have a sex drive, I like men, and I want to be sexual. I hold on to the idea of what sex 'could' be like, or 'should' be like; or even, in times of true optimism, what it 'will' be like. I have never relinquished this hope, this desire" [1].

Mary has tried everything to rid herself of this terrible pain. She talks about her years in denial, her adherence to techniques that put mind over matter, and a whole load of therapy, none of which brought any satisfaction. This led to "more insidious strategies: drinking, drugs, full-body detachment. Along the way, you have infused this cocktail with plenty of self-loathing, guilt, overwhelming sadness, and, increasingly, a sense of total despair" [1].

As her psyche was overwhelmed by the descending spiral of unrelenting pain, she saw her life ruthlessly pass her by. Her friends were buying wonderful new homes, preparing to get married, or expecting another baby. After countless failed relationships and years of pain, Mary found her emotional self at the bottom of the heap. She struggled with these feelings as she lay "on an examination table, with a doctor's hand all the way inside your vagina, massaging the walls of your pelvic floor" [1]. But Mary is quick to point out that her physical therapist was highly professional and listened to her concerns carefully before conducting a physical examination. At her first appointment with the physiotherapist, they told her "I think I can help you, but you have to be prepared to do the work" [1].

Over the next six weeks, she received two forms of treatment, namely, massage and biofeedback. Both of these help sufferers learn how to relax and get their vaginal muscles to act normally. Mary started to check her pelvic floor frequently, as advised by her doctor; yet most of the time, she found it clenched in a protective manner. As she put all her focus into relaxing it, things started improving, all be it marginally [1].

This turned Mary's life around, as it gave her the hope she had never thought possible. "More than anything else, the growing sense of awareness and acceptance is changing my relationship to the pain and to my vagina. The pervasive feeling of helplessness surrounding a taboo topic is falling away" [1].

After the six-week treatment period came to an end, another journey lay ahead. Mary's physiotherapist told her that she had more than just a muscular problem, and referred her to the Center for Vulvovaginal Disorders to meet with the head physician [1].

The following day, Mary went home to celebrate Christmas with her family. While the rest of her relatives were having fun in one room, she had a heart-to-heart with her mother in the dining room. It was here that Mary suddenly found herself opening up about her nightmare for the first time, fighting back tears. Her mother instinctively wrapped her arms around her, saying, "Why didn't you ever tell me? You can't do everything alone" [1]. Mary remembers "in that moment, so many walls between my mother and me came tumbling down. It is the true beginning of letting go" [1].

A few weeks after Christmas, Mary went to her appointment at the Center for Vulvovaginal Disorders. Recalling her emotions at the time, she says "I am tightly wound, equal parts hopeful and skeptical" [1].

Then, to her astonishment, after they arrive in the examination room, the doctor gives Mary a mirror to take an up-close and personal look at her vagina. He then informs her that she is in complete control of what is going to take place. Looking at her vagina this way, something sparked. Mary "had the stunning realization that this thing was mine and that I was solely in control. That this part of me was beautiful and worthy of love" [1].

She advises "Looking at your vagina isn't all that convenient, and I'd even go so far as to say it can be slightly terrifying, but I'd be remiss not to recommend that every woman should spend some time with a hand mirror and her most precious self" [1].

This realization was followed by a second revelation. When the specialist conducted the physical exam, Mary was shocked to find out that the pain which had caused her so much trauma was localized. Restricted to a relatively small region named the vulvar vestibule around the opening of her vagina.

She was then told what she should have been told right from the beginning "I had been born with over 300 times the normal nerve endings at the entrance to my vagina. Instead of sending a signal to the brain that I was being touched, the nerves were instead telling my brain that I was being burned and stabbed" [1]. This condition, which is a form of vulvodynia, is called congenital neuroproliferative vestibulodynia [1].

"I am very emotional as we discuss treatment options" [1]. Mary finally faced her moment of truth as the doctor talked through treatment options. He said "It's really very simple, we remove the bad skin and replace it with healthy skin. After six to eight weeks, you'll be back to work" [1].

But was it all too good to be true? Firstly, the doctor discussed the potential risks the surgery carries, then gave Mary the low down about his patients' success rates, which were very high. He then explained about alternatives to surgery, such as hormone treatments and anti-depressants [1]. The doctor said that these alternatives "may help as a 'patch,' but could never correct the root issue" [1]. Yet the idea of surgery seemed extreme and expensive to Mary [1].

Then her doctor asked her an unexpected question "Do you want children?" [1]. Finding a croaky voice amid her tears, she said yes. "Then you shouldn't wait too much longer," her doctor said. "Talk it over with friends and family. And don't stay away too long" [1].

Leaving the office, Mary was conflicted. She was over-the-moon at having finally received an explanation of her condition, but found it hard to contemplate the idea of surgery. Ultimately, she decided to book the operation for the following December, which was almost 12 months away. That gave her enough time and space to work toward her goal [1].

That December, accompanied by her mother, Mary went in for the procedure. She spent the following two months taking it easy and recuperating. During the healing process, Mary remembers, "I feel like a caterpillar in my cocoon, waiting, changing, transforming. Not just physically, but emotionally as well. I go through a very dark period, but as I begin to heal, a great hope surges through me" [1].

As time healed the emotional and physical wounds of the surgery, and the painful ring of fire around her vagina disappeared, Mary felt like a completely different woman. Eight weeks after the procedure, she once again used a mirror. While her vagina looked slightly different, it was still beautiful. At her first follow-up appointment since the surgery, her doctor "inserts two fingers into my new vagina; I sit up incredulously. There's no pain! Suddenly, tears of joy run down my cheeks and cover my face" [1].

Half a year later, and Mary is totally free of pain.

"If I have learned one thing throughout this process, it's that speaking up about something that is bothering you is always a step in the right direction" [1]. She encourages others to never throw the towel in, but to remain engaged and active on their personal pathway to well-being. "You may have to try many things, but each thing will lead you one step closer to your solution" [1].

Speaking Up Boldly

It's only thanks to sufferers like Mary and the others, who have freely written about their physical and emotional suffering, that the truth about vulvodynia is finally coming out. Thanks to the stories of these women and others, fellow sufferers can find strength, and the rest of the world can begin to fully understand and acknowledge this painful, misunderstood condition.

Chapter 29

Organizations, Support Groups, and Online Health Communities (OHC) for Women with Vulvodynia and Vulvar Pain

Support groups, forums, and healthcare organizations can help you better understand and manage your vulvodynia. The good news is that while vulvodynia is still largely misunderstood, there are a significant number of support groups and resources available. This chapter is a guide to these many resources, presented alphabetically by country and social media platform. Descriptions for each resource are based on the information provided by each.

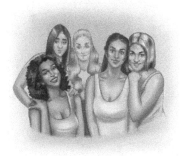

Organizations, support groups, and online health communities (OHC) allow you to discuss and share your experience with others who have the same condition. You might find it easier to discuss sensitive subjects with these people who understand what you are going through, rather than with your family members or friends. Additionally, it helps you feel less alone to know that other people have experienced the same things as you. In fact, peer support has been shown to increase knowledge, self-confidence, and self-care [1].

However, as you engage with these resources, keep in mind that support groups and OHCs should not take the place of medical care or therapy. It's still essential to seek help from a suitably experienced doctor in order to manage your condition.

Argentina

ARACI Asociación Rosarina Afectados Cistitis Intersticial

http://www.araci.org.ar/

https://www.youtube.com/user/LILIARACI/feed

"...the site of ARACI- Rosarina Association of Affected of CI-ARGENTINA, Non-profit Civil Entity that has as its objectives the technical-legal recognition of the pathology we represent, in the National Health System and the dissemination of the disease at all levels: Medical Community, Health Organizations, Population."

Contact for support group meeting details:

Liliana Bacchi, President
menadel_dan@ hotmail.com
0341-4644164
Dorrego 3857-DTO.1
2000 Rosario, Argentina

Australia

The Australian and New Zealand Vulvovaginal Society

http://anzvs.org/

The Australian and New Zealand Vulvovaginal Society (ANZVS) represents gynecologists, dermatologists, pathologists, GPs, sexual health physicians and allied health professionals that have a professional interest in vulvar diseases.

GAIN Inc. Gynaecological Awareness Information Network

https://www.gain.org.au/

GAIN is a not-for-profit organization run by volunteers who dedicate their time to creating a world where every woman has the opportunity, knowledge, confidence and support to obtain optimal gynecological and sexual health.

Pelvic Pain Foundation of Australia

https://www.pelvicpain.org.au/

The Pelvic Pain Foundation of Australia is a not-for-profit organization formed to build a healthier and more productive community by improving the quality of life of people with pelvic pain. We realize that pelvic pain affects many girls, women and men of all ages, ethnicities, and social backgrounds. We aim to minimize the suffering and burden of pelvic pain on individuals, their families and the community through awareness, education, funding, support, and research. This website provides information for those affected by pelvic pain, their families, and their health care providers, regardless of income, location, or access to services.

Vulvodynia Sisters Australia

https://www.facebook.com/groups/1286462514781184/ (Private group)

This is a group for women dealing with vulvodynia, vulvar vestibulitis and dyspareunia in Australia. Share your story, ask questions, and discuss medical professionals and care in Australia.

Bolivia

La Paz IC Support Group

Contact Maria Eulalia Anker
eulalia@ceibo.
entelnet.bo
5912-2712761

Canada

Pelvic Health Solutions

https://pelvichealthsolutions.ca/

Pelvic Health Solutions is an evidence-based teaching company that was founded in 2010 by Nelly Faghani and Carolyn Vandyken, out of the need to develop pelvic health resources in Ontario, an under serviced health concern in this province. Since the inception of our teaching company, pelvic health physiotherapy has blossomed from a handful of physiotherapists to well over 300 therapists now rostered with the Ontario College of Physiotherapists

Chile

Sociedad Chilena De Uroginecología Y Piso Pélvico (SODUP)

(Chilean Society of Urogynecology and Pelvic Floor)

http://sodup.cl/?avia_forced_reroute=1

We are a multidisciplinary group from the different areas of health, focused on the study and management of the Pelvic Floor.

Mission:

Facilitate access to information among partners, other institutions, organizations, and patients.

Favor scientific and academic spaces to share clinical experiences and improve the knowledge of its partners in this area.

Promote the formation of Multidisciplinary teams to deliver comprehensive responses to patients with different pathologies of the Pelvic Floor.

Vision:

Position itself as a multidisciplinary scientific society present and at the forefront, being a national and international benchmark, in the public and private spheres to improve the daily life of patients.

Denmark

Danish Vulvodynia Association

https://vulvodyni.info/

Danish Vulvodynia Association is a patient association. We will focus on the hidden pain. Vulvodynia feels like a burning sensation in the abdomen. Many women with vulvodynia experience pain during sex, and intercourse may be impossible.

Viden om vulvodyni

https://www.facebook.com/groups/1374874716087728/ (Private group)

This group is about vulvodynia (abdominal pain in women)

The group is for women who are directly affected by the disorder, their partners, and professionals. It is permissible to ask questions about the disorder and its mental and physical challenges, share its history, share treatment or lecture etc. If you are unsure what to do, send a message to the administrator. The group is set up with the aim of disseminating more knowledge about vulvodynia - and not least treatment options. There are up to 40,000-60,000 women suffering from vulvodynia in Denmark, and for many this means that it is impossible to perform intercourse due to pain in the abdomen. Much knowledge is still lacking in this area, and I hope that this group can help relevant professionals become more competent and help the women and partners affected by vulvodynia. So here you have the opportunity as a woman, or partner to ask questions, and as a professional to offer her knowledge, therapy, or treatment. Success stories on treatment are very welcome!

NOTE: vaginism, lichen sclerosis and dyspareunia are certainly also relevant in the group and very welcome.

There is also a support group, which is ONLY for women with vulvodynia, and their partners (i.e., not professionals), where you can support and guide each other: https://www.facebook.com/groups/99117664922/

Finland

Gynekologinen potilasjärjestö Korento ry. The Gynecological Patient Association Korento

https://korento.fi/

The Finnish patient association for people with vulvodynia, endometriosis, adenomyosis and PCOS offers face to face support groups as well as online peer support such as discussion groups and chats. Korento also offers up-to-date information on the diseases and syndromes it represents. Another goal is to raise awareness of menstruation and which symptoms are typical and when to seek help from healthcare professionals. The association has developed Moona Symptom Diary, a mobile app for monitoring menstrual cycle and symptoms related to it. Moona is a helpful tool for anyone but especially for people with a gynecological condition or syndrome. At the time of writing Moona is only available in Finland, but Korento is currently working towards making it globally available.

Elämää vulvodynian kanssa
https://www.hyvakysymys.fi/keskusteluryhmat/elamaa-vulvodynian-kanssa/
A closed discussion group maintained by Korento for everyone who is affected by vulvodynia, i.e. those who live with or suspect themselves of vulvodynia.

Vulvodynia Suomi (Vulvodynia Finland)
https://www.facebook.com/groups/vulvodyniasuomi/ (Private group)
The group is a closed peer support group maintained by Korento and intended for everyone living with or suspecting vulvodynia. The group is moderated by volunteer members of the organization who also participate in the discussions as themselves, unless they make it clear that they are acting in a maintenance role.

Please answer the question asked in connection with the request to join, only then will you be accepted into the group. People added by others are not directly accepted into the group, they also must answer questions. The purpose of the group is to share proven self-care methods and support others during difficult days. General discussion on the topic e.g., expert caregivers, diet, supplements, and sexuality.

Germany

Vulvodynia Support Deutschland

https://www.facebook.com/groups/783132358759557/   (Private group)

This group is intended to be a forum for exchange. As a sufferer, I received a lot of support and information from American groups. In this group, those affected can share their experiences, give advice, and make recommendations. Because in dealing with vulvodynia and vestibulodynia, I learned above all that you yourself must become the best expert here. Doctors and therapists are also welcomed to join the group and support them in the exchange.

India

Chronic Pain India

https://chronicpainindia.com/

https://www.facebook.com/chronicpainindia/

https://twitter.com/chronicpainind?lang=en

https://in.pinterest.com/chronicpainindia/

https://www.instagram.com/chronicpainindia/

A Charitable Trust trying to raise awareness in India about various chronic pain conditions and chronic illness which are usually invisible to naked eyes.

Vulvodynia is listed in "the list of conditions, we at Chronic Pain India are trying to raise awareness for" (https://chronicpainindia.com/conditions/).

Pelvic Pain India

https://www.pelvicpainindia.com/

https://www.facebook.com/pelvicpainindia/ (listed as 'Nonprofit Organization')

https://www.instagram.com/pelvicpainindia/

Pelvic pain is of the least talked about and undertreated medical conditions as people find it hard to talk about. This group is aimed at helping and guiding people with pelvic pain.

Interstitial Cystitis India

http://www.interstitialcystitisinindia.org/

https://www.facebook.com/groups/1803197073289466/ (Private group)

https://www.youtube.com/channel/UC6kTJ2A2-CUGZOLPATGOdyQ

We at Interstitial Cystitis India are here to help patients suffering from Interstitial Cystitis in India and neighboring countries. We are a group of IC patients who have come together to help other IC patients suffering from this disease. ICI is a non-profit voluntary organization which promotes knowledge and awareness of interstitial cystitis (IC), bladder pain syndrome (BPS), painful bladder syndrome (PBS), hypersensitive bladder (HSB), chronic pelvic pain (CPP) and associated disorders among patients, patient support groups, health professionals, medical practitioners, doctors, medical students, caregivers, the family of patients, health authorities, legislatures, and the public. No salaries or remuneration are paid to members who work on an entirely voluntary basis. We are in the process of getting registered.

Ireland

Vulvodynia Support Ireland

https://www.facebook.com/groups/1381996548482415/ (Private group)

Supporting and exchanging ideas with women from Ireland who suffer with vulvodynia.

Italy

Associazione VulvodiniaPuntoInfo ONLUS

https://www.vulvodiniapuntoinfo.com/

https://www.facebook.com/groups/VulvodiniaPuntoInfoONLUS/
(Private group)

Non-profit organization of social utility. Since 2010 the voice of women with vulvodynia/Vulvo-Vestibular Syndrome.

Netherlands

Vulvodynie Nl

https://www.facebook.com/groups/1727079760863579/ (Private group)

This group is for every woman who has or has had vulvodynia, vaginismus, vestibular vulvitis (also called focal vulvitis), dyspareunia and other related diagnoses.

New Zealand

Vulvodynia Support New Zealand

http://vulvodynia.org.nz/

Vulvodynia Support NZ. This site is intended as a resource for women with vulvodynia and their partners. If you have vulvodynia, or think that you might, this site is for you. If your partner has vulvodynia, this site is for you. Vulvodynia is not well-known, even in medical circles. Even within gynecology, it is hard to get a mention. Women with vulvodynia deserve support and respect. We deserve effective, accessible treatment. Most of all we deserve not to be left thinking that we are the only one.

Vulvodynia Support NZ

https://www.facebook.com/groups/240954829363720/ (Private group)

I have created this group so that women in NZ (although we do welcome members from everywhere!) can easily get in touch with each other to provide support, discuss and learn more about Vulvodynia, Vestibulodynia etc. If you would like further support/info, please email us at vulvodyniasupport@hotmail.co.nz

Peru

Dispareunia Peru

https://es.groups.yahoo.com/neo/groups/dispareunia_peru/info

Support group dedicated to men and women living in Peru and for whom sexual intercourse is painful.

Spain

Dedicado a mujeres que padecen de dolor vulvar (Dedicated to women suffering from vulvar pain)

https://es.groups.yahoo.com/neo/groups/vulvodinia/info
(Restricted group)

Vulvodynia is the generic name that refers to the sensation of burning, stinging or pain in the vulva, in the vaginal vestibule or in the vagina. This group is intended as a place where women who suffer or have suffered from vulvodynia (in its categories: dysesthesia or vestibulitis) can share their concerns and experiences. Doctors, researchers, family, and friends are also welcome.

Blog para mujeres que padecen de vulvodinia

http://vulvodinia.blogspot.com/

For women, friends, doctors, nurses, family members and people interested in learning more about this painful physical condition.

South America

Asociación Latinoamericana de Piso Pélvico (ALAPP)

Latin American Pelvic Floor Association

https://alapp.org/

https://www.facebook.com/somosalapp/

https://twitter.com/ALAPPnews

https://www.instagram.com/somosalapp/

https://www.youtube.com/channel/UC60i6zAvLyV-7kWC7qtxc2Q

The Latin American Pelvic Floor Association is a non-profit association founded in 2015, whose main objectives are the training, dissemination and research of all aspects related to the area of voiding, anorectal and pelvic floor dysfunction.

See the website for Friendly Societies https://alapp.org/sociedades-amigas/.

United Kingdom (UK)

The British Pain Society

www.britishpainsociety.org/

This UK society comprises a professional alliance which promotes the management and understanding of pain to patients.

BSSVD British Society for the Study of Vulvovaginal Diseases

https://bssvd.org/

This UK organization offers patients a plethora of useful information about vulvar conditions.

International Pelvic Pain Society (IPPS)

https://www.pelvicpain.org/

In 1995 a group of physicians met to discuss their common interest in addressing a gap in chronic pelvic pain research, diagnostics, support, and treatment. After two years, the International Pelvic Pain Society (IPPS) was incorporated to serve as a forum for professional and public education. Since then, the IPPS has grown to include gynecologists, urologists, gastroenterologists, physicians, physical and occupational therapists, psychologists, social workers and other health professionals committed to a biopsychosocial and interdisciplinary approach for the treatment of conditions associated with chronic pelvic pain.

@PelvicPainOrg

https://twitter.com/pelvicpainorg

The International Pelvic Pain Society's mission is to improve diagnosis and treatment of pelvic pain, helping to improve the lives of suffering patients.

Pelvic Guru Academy for Health and Fitness Professionals

https://pelvicguru.com/

At Pelvic Guru, we are building a trusted global network connecting pelvic health professionals in the medical, sexual health, women's health, and fitness fields with community members. We know that so many people are dealing with pelvic pain, pregnancy and postpartum conditions, reproductive and genital cancers, leaking with activity, and so much more; and are seeking help!

https://www.facebook.com/groups/pelvicgurumentoring   (Private group)

For health and fitness professionals only. Find out the latest info on the upcoming courses and mentoring opportunities from Pelvic Guru Academy. Connect with many professionals about all things pelvic health.

Pelvic Pain Support Network

https://www.pelvicpain.org.uk/

This UK support network is a patient led organization with a board of trustees. All the latter are either carers or patients. It offers advocacy, information, and support to sufferers of pelvic pain, as well as their carers and families. Further, the network delivers and promotes educational sessions on pelvic pain.

Pudendal Neuralgia and Pelvic Pain UK

https://www.facebook.com/groups/1614073482191502/ (Private group)

Welcome to Pudendal Neuralgia and Pelvic Pain UK. Although we are sorry you need to join this group, we hope we will be of help. It is a group for both sexes. This group has been set up primarily for anyone living in the UK. We all need to be able to talk about the facilities and doctors we have in the UK. However, anyone suffering from Pudendal and Pelvic pain is welcome.

Pudendal Neuralgia and Vulvodynia UK

https://www.facebook.com/groups/1109555252408851/

A transitional group which allows ladies to join a private Facebook group once the administrator of the group has had contact with them. As the official group's members want it to remain private, we can't provide details here, but if you follow the above link to the group and, if necessary, sign up with Facebook, you can contact the administrator for details on how to join the group itself.

Support for UK women with vulval pain

https://groups.yahoo.com/neo/groups/UKVulvalPain/info

Email support group for UK women suffering from vulvar pain, vulvodynia, vulvar vestibulitis, lichen sclerosis, and other vulvar problems.

Vulval Pain Partners

https://uk.groups.yahoo.com/neo/groups/vulval_pain_partners/info

A UK support group for partners of women with vulvar pain syndromes such as vulvodynia, vestibulodynia, lichen sclerosis and PNE (pudendal nerve entrapment).

The Vulval Pain Society

http://www.vulvalpainsociety.org

This British society provides information on all areas related to vulvar pain. Moreover, it works to protect and promote the mental and physical health of vulvar pain sufferers through the provision of practical advice, education, and support. It also has an extensive list of support groups in the UK.

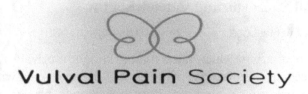

Vulvodynia UK

https://www.facebook.com/groups/vulvodyniauk/ (Private group)

This is a support group for women who have vulvodynia, those who think they may have it and those who experience any type of vulvar pain. I have called it Vulvodynia UK simply because I would like to meet women in my area/country who have this condition. Having vulvodynia has, at times, made my life very difficult but not impossible. There are ways of living with this condition and life is to be enjoyed not endured! Please join us if you would like some support and advice with lots of laughs along the way. Feel free to join and add any material which will help us in our quest to cope with this condition.

United Kingdom (UK) by Region

Bristol Vulval Health Support Group

https://sites.google.com/view/bristolvhsg

This group aims to support women with a range of vulvar health conditions, including lichen sclerosis, vulvodynia, vaginismus, and other conditions that may or may not be formally diagnosed.

Cornwall Lichen Sclerosus and Vulvodynia Support Group

Call 07547 210293

Cross Pennines Vulval Pain Support Group

https://sites.google.com/site/cpvpsg/

We offer support to women who suffer with vulvar conditions such as vulvodynia, vestibulodynia (vestibulitis), vaginismus, lichen sclerosis, interstitial cystitis, and vulvar eczema. The group is active in Yorkshire and the North West.

The London Vulval Pain Support Group

https://sites.google.com/site/londonvpsg/home

We provide confidential support and advice for women in the London area who suffer from vulvar pain.

Manchester Vulval Support Network

https://www.mvsn.co.uk/

MVSN was created in 2015 by a team of patient representatives, two Consultant Gynecologists and a specialist Nurse. The group was created to meet the needs of women with vulvar pain issues in the North West of England. It was recognized that there was a lack of face-to-face support for what can be a challenging and isolating condition

Sandyford Girls Vulval Pain Support Group

For more information, please contact Sandyford Central on 0141 232 8414

Somerset Vulvodynia Network

Call the group administrator on 07307 633820 or email at vulvodyniasomerset@gmail.com

Welsh Marches Vulval Pain Support Group

https://groups.io/g/wmvpsg

This group has been created to help and support women with vulvar pain. Vulvar pain can affect all aspects of daily life, emotionally as well as physically. We do not give diagnosis or offer medical advice. We are here to help fellow sufferers, talk through issues and suggest ways of relieving symptoms.

United States (US)

American Chronic Pain Association

https://www.theacpa.org/

Since 1980, the ACPA has offered peer support and education in pain management skills to people with pain, family and friends, and health care professionals. The information and tools on our site can help you to better understand your pain and work more effectively with your health care team toward a higher quality of life.

Chronic Pain Support Group

https://www.facebook.com/groups/11864244228/ (Private group)

Finding Pelvic Sanity - Pelvic Health Support

https://www.facebook.com/groups/findingpelvicsanity/ (Private group)

Practical, positive information for those with pelvic pain or pelvic health issues to help you find lasting relief. Moderated by the experts at PelvicSanity physical therapy, every member has made a commitment to support each other with encouragement, helpful questions, and by sharing their experiences.

https://www.instagram.com/pelvicsanity/

https://linktr.ee/pelvicsanity

{Ties to https://www.pelvicsanity.com/}

The International Society for the Study of Vulvovaginal Disease (ISSVD)

https://www.issvd.org/

The World's Number 1 Resource for Vulvar Education and Research.

The National Vulvodynia Association

https://www.nva.org/

This leading US association offers detailed information on current treatments, and suspected causes of vulvodynia. It also provides important resources, learning tools, and the latest research results on this complex disease.

It emphasizes a coordinated interdisciplinary approach to sufferers' medical care; and works to educate women about vulvodynia, thus empowering them to make informed choices about different treatments.

It also inspires women to tackle the emotional and physical components of vulvodynia, through the development of self-help strategies. Further, the association aims to promote a supportive family environment by educating patients' loved ones. A comprehensive list of support groups in the U.S. and Canada can also be found on the site.

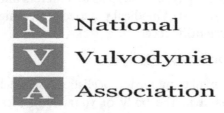

Painful Sex & Chronic Pelvic Pain Conditions (by PainDownThere)

https://www.facebook.com/groups/paindownthere/

This group is moderated by a women's health and functional nutrition coach. PainDownThere.com's Robert Echenberg, MD and physical therapist, Karen Liberi MS, MPT, WCS are also consulted on questions and discussions within this group.

The Patty Brisben Foundation for Women's Sexual Health

http://pattybrisbenfoundation.org/national-vulvodynia-association/

The Patty Brisben Foundation has funded a national vulvodynia "outcomes treatment registry," a research study focused on finding the best course of treatment for patients suffering from vulvovaginal pain. We have also supported an online tutorial for women with vulvodynia. The online tutorial has brought awareness to the under-researched and typically little-discussed topic of vaginal pain disorders.

Pudendal Help

http://www.pudendalhope.info/

This international organization offers information and support to patients who are suffering from pudendal nerve entrapment (PNE), pudendal neuralgia (PN), or pudendal neuropathy (PN).

The VP Foundation

http://www.thevpfoundation.org/

The VP (Vulvar Pain) Foundation was established in 1992 as a nonprofit organization to end the isolation of women suffering from vulvar pain and related disorders (fibromyalgia, interstitial cystitis, irritable bowel). The Foundation's purposes are to give reliable information, hope, safety, and success to sufferers and their families, to advance the standard of medical practice in treating the syndrome, and to promote scientific research.

Vulvar Pain Forum (VPF)

To join, send an email to majordomo@lists.jabberwocky.com with the following command in the body of your email message: subscribe vulvarpainforum

Description   from:
http://www.vulvalpainsociety.org/vps/index.php/vulval-pain-support-groups/outside-the-uk

Vulvovaginal Disorders

http://vulvovaginaldisorders.com

This US organization offers an algorithm for basic diagnosis and treatment. Its complete women's health care for vulvovaginal offers various resources including a free learning program, and patient handouts.

United States (US) by State

National Vulvodynia Association

Support Contacts and Support Group Meetings

https://www.nva.org/for-patients/support-services/

It is important to be able to talk with other women about the physical symptoms of vulvodynia and related emotional issues. Many women find that speaking to others who have vulvodynia is both a good source of information and the best way to overcome the emotional isolation that may result from having this disorder. The NVA has identified the below support groups and email contacts for those who choose this option. Please note that some of the below listed groups may be working to build a support group and, therefore, may not always be actively meeting. The groups may also take breaks from meeting on occasion, and some groups may also meet more often than others.

Sun City (Arizona)

Contact: Randi; courtice@cox.net

Upcoming Meetings: Please email for information on other upcoming meetings. Location: Please email for specifics and directions.

California-

Contact: Cheryl; jmorris4550-nva@yahoo.com

Upcoming Meetings: No meetings. Email support only. Special interest in post-menopausal issues and lichen sclerosus.

Location: California

San Francisco (California)

Contact: Terry; tsbohrer@yahoo.com

Upcoming Meetings: Please email for more information on upcoming meetings.

Location: Please email for specifics and directions.

Middletown (Connecticut)

Contact: ctpelvic@gmail.com

Upcoming Meetings: Please email for information on upcoming meetings.

Location: Please email for specifics and directions.

Royal Oak (Michigan)

Contact: The Women's Urology and Pelvic Health Center; 248-898-0898

Upcoming Meetings:

The Pelvic Pain Support Group of Beaumont Hospital helps women with pelvic pain (including but not limited to IC, vulvar pain, pelvic floor dysfunction, among other forms of uro-genital pain) get the support of others with similar problems, and encourages participants to take active, positive steps toward coping. Staff from the Women's Urology and Pelvic Health Center will facilitate the group. The group meets monthly and is free of charge. Meetings will be held on Thursdays, approximately once per month from 11:30 am to 1:00 pm.

Location:

Women's Urology and Pelvic Health Center

2 South, Beaumont Hospital

3601 W. 13 Mile Road

Royal Oak, MI 48073

Saginaw (Michigan)

Contact: Kathy; adatte5689@charter.net

Upcoming Meetings: No Meetings, email support only.

Location: Saginaw, MI

New York (NY)

Contact: Judy; drjudysi@gmail.com

Upcoming Meetings: No meetings, email support only. Special interest in post-menopausal issues.

Location: New York City, NY

Rochester (New York)

Contact: Katy Wright; nvarochester@gmail.com

Upcoming Meetings: No Meetings, email support only.

Location: Rochester, NY

Tulsa (Oklahoma)

Contact: Jodi; jodilyncole@gmail.com ; 918-520-1752

Upcoming Meetings: Please email or call for information on upcoming meetings.

Location: Tulsa Spine & Rehab, 3345 S Harvard Avenue #101 Tulsa. Please email or call for specifics and directions.

Portland (Oregon)

Contact: Krista; sexualpainmatters@gmail.com

Upcoming Meetings: No meetings currently, email support only.

Location: Portland, OR

Kent (Washington)

Contact: Gerry; carrickrock@yahoo.com ; 206-310-2540

Upcoming Meetings: No meetings, email, phone, and text support only.

Location: Kent, WA

California

Bloomin' Uterus Endometriosis Support: San Diego and SoCal

San Diego, CA

https://bloominuterus.com/support-group/

I was diagnosed with Stage IV Endometriosis in June of 2014. And I have since been searching for a community support group where other San Diego-area EndoSisters could come together to assist one another in an exchange of information and emotional support. I was unable to find one but did learn that several of my close friends also suffered from Endometriosis. Having not found a community group, we created one and our first meeting took place in January 2015. And we have continued to meet every month since, and our numbers have continued to grow.

Come share with us. Or just come and listen. Sometimes we do not even talk about Endo at all. It is a completely stress-free environment: no expectations, no judgments. We are simply here for each other.

We will never seek to profit from this. We will freely share anything we have learned with each other.

Self-promotion, sales of items, fundraisers, and business networking are prohibited from these meetings. Any support groups, meet-ups, or walks we organize will never charge admission or registration. Nor will they be a platform for those who seek to self-promote their interests and products for profit, popularity, political, or personal gain. You are not a target demographic to us to profit from or use for self-advancement. We are sisters and will do for each other as sisters do. This is our Code.

San Jose Healing Chronic Pelvic Pain Meetup Group

San Jose, CA (Public group)

https://www.meetup.com/San-Jose-Healing-Chronic-Pelvic-Pain-Meetup-Group/

This is a group for anyone interested in findings solutions to live beyond chronic pelvic pain. I started this group to meet other women in search of solutions. Let's meet, share, and learn!

Florida

Pelvic Pain or Bladder Issues Support Group

Volusia County, FL

Pelvic Pain or Bladder Issues Support Group: 386-492-3115.

Pelvic Pain Support Group

Boca Raton Regional Hospital), Boca Raton, FL

https://www.brrh.com/Services/Classes-Events-Support-Groups/Drummond-Rehabilitation-Institute.aspx

This lecture series and support group provided by the Barbara C. Gutin Center for Pelvic Health is designed for individuals living with pelvic and abdominal pain and dysfunction. Meetings feature a guest speaker who will focus on helpful topics and allow for open discussion. The group meets on various Wednesdays from 6pm-7pm at Lynn Women's Health & Wellness Institute.

Women's Pelvic Pain Support Group

Hollywood, FL (Public group)

https://www.meetup.com/PelvicPainSupport/

A group for women with pelvic pain. Online support groups can be valuable, but we want to give each other the personal support and connection that a friend who truly understands what you are going through can provide. Meetings will be led by a Doctor of Physical Therapy, who specializes in women's health. We will meet, share, and learn. Most importantly, we want these meetings to be positive, uplifting events. Often the weight of our own pain combined with the stories of others can make us feel worse instead of better! We will strive to uplift each other, providing support and actionable information at each meeting.

Maryland

Maryland Vulvar Pain Support Group

Crofton, MD

Maryland Vulvar Pain Support Group meets the third Saturday of each month at 1:30 p.m. at the Crofton Library. 410-721-1583.

Massachusetts

Meetup Groups: Pelvic Floor Dysfunction for Women Boston

Boston, MA (Private Group)

https://www.meetup.com/Pelvic-Floor-Dysfunction-for-Women-Boston/

1. The purpose of the group is to meet other women struggling with pelvic floor dysfunction and disorders in a private setting. We will have icebreaker coffee meetups and eventually meet at a community center room for more privacy since the topics can be sensitive in nature. For example, the pelvic floor is responsible for bladder, bowel, and sexual function, most of which are taboo to discuss in society.

2. Who should Join? Women only (those with female sex organs) who are diagnosed with or are questioning a diagnosis of pelvic floor dysfunction/disorders.

3. While we are primarily a support group, I will also make sure that what we discuss is scientifically accurate. This will be a sister group to the Facebook group "Pelvic Floor Dysfunction Boston - women only!" which already has over 100 infographics and anatomy photographs of the female pelvis. We will share information on providers, articles, recommendations, and personal experiences. Everything that is said in the group stays in the group. Privacy is of utmost importance

Michigan

Women Coping Support Group

Beaumont Hospital, Royal Oak, MI

https://www.beaumont.org/services/urology/womens-urology-center/women-coping-support-group

For women with interstitial cystitis, vulvar pain and other uro-genital pain problems.

The Women Coping Pelvic Pain Support Group helps women with pelvic pain get the support of others with similar problems, and encourages participants to take active, positive steps toward coping. Staff from the Women's Urology Center will facilitate the group. We ask that attendees be considerate of each other and refrain from wearing scented lotions and perfumes to these meetings as we would like to maintain a scent-free environment for people with sensitivities/allergies.

New York

Brooklyn Interstitial Cystitis Meetup Group

Brooklyn, NY (Public group)

https://www.meetup.com/Brooklyn-Interstitial-Cystitis-Meetup-Group/

By creating this group my hope is to establish a local community where we can leave our apartments and not only meet, but also form bonds with others suffering from IC. This group is open to all who have IC, and their significant others who would like to acquire more information about this chronic illness.

Since a lot of us have difficulty with foods and alcohol, I figured Coffee Shops serving tea assortments would be a good place to start. During our meetups, you can expect sharing stories and bonding over tea, and eventually I would like to host fun activities like bowling or picnic potlucks with IC friendly foods. Hope to see you at the meetups.

Long Island Women's Health Healing Group

Babylon, NY (Private group)

https://www.meetup.com/Long-Island-Womens-Health-Healing-Group/

A place for women to get together to share ways to heal women's health issues including pelvic pain, incontinence, vulvodynia, fibromyalgia, painful breasts/ implants/ reductions/ mastectomy. For more information, please visit:

http://www.chronicpainpt.com

http://www.fertilitylongisland.com.

New York Pelvic Floor Health Meetup

New York, NY (Public group)

https://www.meetup.com/New-York-Pelvic-Floor-Health-Meetup/

For women and men interested in learning about pelvic floor health and preventative measures they can take to prevent pelvic floor dysfunction such as stress incontinence, urge incontinence, pelvic pain, erectile dysfunction, painful intercourse, chronic constipation, fecal incontinence, and pelvic organ prolapse.

Pelvic Pain Support Group for Women

New York, NY (Private group)

https://www.meetup.com/Pelvic-Pain-Support-Group-for-Women-NYC/

The Pelvic Pain Support Group for Women NYC is for women living with pelvic pain looking to connect with others, share their stories, if they choose, and elevate pelvic pain as an issue that should be prioritized in the women's public health area. Pelvic pain can impact women of varying ages, race and ethnic identities, and cultural backgrounds. This group aims to offer women living with pelvic pain a sense of community, a resource for information and services, and an opportunity to speak up and share their own stories.

Whether you are experiencing pelvic pain for the first time, are a survivor of sexual assault, or have lived with chronic pain for several years, you are invited to join the community.

Vaginismus Support Group

Maze Women's Sexual Health, New York, NY; Purchase, NY

https://www.mazewomenshealth.com/forums/forum/vaginismus/

Maze advocates diagnosis of and treatment for the physical causes of female sexual dysfunction, as well as any underlying psychological influences, by integrating education and psychological counseling with medical techniques specifically to help you achieve a full and satisfying sex life.

Vulvar Pain Support Group

Cheektowaga, NY (outside Buffalo)

Vulvar Pain Support Group will meet in St. Luke's Lutheran Church, 900 Maryvale Drive, Cheektowaga. For information, call Ellen at 825-4870.

North Carolina

Chronic Pain Support Group of Charlotte

https://www.facebook.com/groups/cpsofcharlotte/

This group is being established to serve and join those who suffer from chronic pain and for those who care for loved one's suffering from chronic pain.

North Dakota

Fargo Moorhead (FM) Pelvic Pain Support Group

West Fargo, ND

https://www.facebook.com/fmpelvicpain/

https://twitter.com/FMPelvicPain

Fargo Moorhead Pelvic Pain Support Group, for those suffering from endometriosis, PCOS, pelvic inflammatory disease, bladder pain, IC, dysmenorrhea, menorrhagia, uterine fibroids, ovarian cysts, IBS, dyspareunia and vaginismus, meets at 6 p.m. at Physical Therapy Wellness Center, 550 13th Ave. E., West Fargo. (218) 790-0432. Call for meeting dates.

Oregon

Pelvic Pain Pals

Eugene, OR

https://www.meetup.com/Pelvic-Pain-Pals/ (Public group)

https://www.facebook.com/groups/376566532943591/about/ (Private group)

This group is for all women who experience chronic pelvic pain— sounds fun right?! 15% of women in the US have some form of chronic pelvic pain for up to 6 months. This includes vulvodynia, endometriosis, interstitial cystitis, ovarian cysts, etc. I want to have a safe group that can openly talk about what we are going through. Let us get together and rant, talk about relationships, talk about what we are doing to heal, and everything in-between.

Vulvar Vestibulitis Support Network

Portland, OR

https://www.facebook.com/groups/198212676858921 (Private group)

https://groups.yahoo.com/neo/groups/vvsn/info (Restricted group)

https://vvssupport.wordpress.com/

The Vulvar Vestibulitis Support Network (formerly NVVO) is committed to the education, healing, and support for women suffering with Vulvar Vestibulitis Syndrome (VVS) and other similar chronic vulvovaginal pain disorders. We are organizing and distributing information and doing presentations to increase awareness about Vulvar Vestibulitis Syndrome locally and its symptoms, treatments, and the stories of us women who survive and thrive through this disorder. We are also advocates of the face to face support group! It has changed the quality of all our lives immeasurably! We would like to help you set one up in your area if you are interested. Our mission is to bring support and relief to women who suffer with chronic vaginal pain.

We are in Portland Oregon. We are looking for new members for our awesome wonderful support group! If you are in a location near us, we would love to meet up with you! Our meetings are usually on Saturdays in SE Portland. We are, however, flexible, and would love to meet other women in the area with this condition.

Our Yahoo online support group is:
http://health.groups.yahoo.com/group/vvsn/ and although we are not as active of a group as others, we welcome new members! We seem to be using Facebook more! We also have a
blog: http://vvssupport.wordpress.com/. Please contact us (or post to the Facebook group) if you have any questions.
vsssupport@gmail.com

Pennsylvania

Interstitial Cystitis/ Pelvic Pain Support Group

The Resiliency Center, Flourtown, PA

https://theresiliencycenter.com/group/interstitial-cystitispelvic-pain-support-group/

Ongoing monthly support and psycho-educational group providing an opportunity to connect with others with Interstitial Cystitis and/or Pelvic Pain symptoms. Share experiences, coping strategies and resources while learning to take care of yourself. Speakers presenting on topics related to Interstitial Cystitis and Pelvic Pain conditions are offered throughout the year.

Pelvic Pain Support Group

Empower Physical Therapy, Exton, PA

https://www.physicaltherapyempower.com/events

This support group is designed for discussion, dialogue and education about pelvic pain and disorders. It is a supportive environment to educate and empower women to utilize holistic treatment methods to manage chronic pain and pelvic related conditions. Your host, Allison Landry, was diagnosed with Vulvodynia and manages chronic pain daily. 2nd Tuesday of each month

Pelvic Pain Support Group

UPMC Susquehanna, Muncy, PA (central Pennsylvania)

https://www.susquehannahealth.org/services/rehabilitation-services/support-groups

If you live with chronic pelvic pain, please join us to meet other women who live with endometriosis, interstitial cystitis, and other pelvic pain conditions. This group offers a supportive and positive experience.

UPMC Susquehanna Muncy; Call (570) 546-4291 for more information or to register.

Texas

Female Sexual Pain Support Group in Austin, TX

The Pathway to Pleasure Collective, Austin, TX

https://www.pathwaytopleasure.com/female-sexual-pain-support-group-austin.html

The Female Sexual Pain Support group is intended to be a sacred space for women to explore their full range of thoughts, feelings and emotions regarding the challenges they are facing with dyspareunia. It is also intended to be a place for you to experience new ways of connecting with your body and your emotions in a way that works with your body's wisdom rather than against it. Oftentimes when there is pain in the body the inclination is to avoid it, to numb it out, and to get away from it. While the roots and causes of dyspareunia are complex and unique to each woman and treatment approaches will vary depending on the type of sexual pain you are experiencing, including the body's innate wisdom is a critical part of any healing process.

And unfortunately, when we do not include the body wisdom in our healing not only do we miss the deeper messages yearning to be acknowledged by our bodies, but we often unintentionally give the pain more strength and power over us. It is only when we fully embrace and unconditionally meet what is exactly the way it is, that we can eventually transform it. This is the paradox of change! And this is the aim of the female sexual pain support group at The Pathway to Pleasure Collective.

Pelvic Pain Support Group

Sullivan Physical Therapy, Austin, TX

Pelvic Pain Support Group 10 to 11:15 am 4131 Spicewood Springs Road Suite M-1 Austin, Texas 78759. RSVP prior to joining the group: brittanyneece@gmail.com or 512-814-6027

Washington

Washington DC NVA Vulvodynia Support Group

Washington, D.C.

Sponsored by National Vulvodynia Association, for women with chronic vulvar pain.

DC Area Group Leader: Kathy, 703-335-8286, Contact_Leader@yahoo.com

Other Organizations and Support Groups

Blogs

Inspire Santé

http://inspiresante.org/

Pelvic pain is common. But it is not normal. You can heal. We want to help. We are a nonprofit that provides advocacy and education for pelvic pain disorders. Click around, learn more, and reach out with questions. We are here to help. Restoring your hope is our mission. We supply the community, inspiration, and education to elevate your healing. Our blog: real stories from real women

Oklahoma Women's IC & Pelvic Pain Support

http://ichopeok.blogspot.com/

Welcome to Oklahoma Women's IC & Chronic Pelvic Pain Support! This blog has been specially created for those suffering from any kind of pelvic pain disorder (i.e. Interstitial Cystitis, CPP, VV, PFD, but not limited to) who are looking for others with similar struggles. Although many posts are focused on IC, you will however find all sorts of great tips on coping with CPP, treatment options, featured guest stories, to yummy recipes that make following the 'IC' diet a breeze.

Vulvodynia Siren

https://vulvodyniasirenblog.wordpress.com/

Managing Female Pain and Health; My experience with pelvic pain and surgery: Vulvodynia/ Vestibulitis & Vestibulectomy

Facebook (Only)

Early Onset Lichen Sclerosis/Sclerosus/vulvodynia Support Group

https://www.facebook.com/groups/218458219352900/ (Private group)

This is a support group for adults who have personally been coping with LS, Vulvodynia, VIN, Vestibulitis, or related conditions from an early age (childhood/ adolescence). It is for patients only, not health professionals, relatives, or researchers. Dealing with chronic vulvar conditions takes is challenging for anyone. Coping with the physical as well as mental and social aspects long term and especially, from formative years, adds extra layers of complexity. Given that this is often still a "taboo" topic to discuss socially and is often (mis) categorized as a "rare" condition, it can be a very isolating and shamed condition, often with few to no spaces to share with others in a similar situation. Early onset sufferers may find it helpful to have a safe space to process feelings internalized from their formative years, and to share continued long term health management strategies, successes, and challenges that may differ from those who were more recently diagnosed as adults.

Fibromialgia E Vulvodinia: Dal Confronto Alla Guarigione

https://www.facebook.com/groups/844906938898486/ (Private group)

A place of refreshment and comparison for those who find themselves having to fight against these two pathologies. Have a good trip and good healing to all!

Interstitial Cystitis and Vulvodynia Support and More

https://www.facebook.com/groups/445818108927920/ (Private group)

My Hiding Place: Support for Christians with Vulvodynia

https://www.facebook.com/groups/1813577425616879/ (Private group)

This group is for Bible-believing, genetic females only. It is a place where we come to share the joy of having a relationship with Christ and the struggle of living with the pain of vulvodynia. It is not for perfect people, rather it is for all repentant sinners who are in Christ. It is a place for honest discussion among Christians who are expected to act like Christians (1 Corinthians 13). We are the body of Christ, and we need each other. Let us support, comfort, acknowledge, exhort, and sharpen (Prov. 27:17) one another as we seek to honor God.

Partners of Vulvodynia

https://www.facebook.com/groups/partnersofvulvodynia/

A private Facebook group for men whose partners suffer from vulvar pain. They say: "This group has been set up for men whose partners are suffering from vulvodynia. It's important that we offer support and help raise awareness around this rare condition." To join the group, sign up with Facebook if you need to, then just follow the above link to the group page and follow the instructions on the page.

Unite per la Vestibolite

https://www.facebook.com/groups/124930100867782/ (Private group)

Association for patients with vulvo-vestibular syndrome (vestibulitis). Administrator: Elisa Marenco, e-mail: elisa.marenco@gmail.com

Vaginismus

https://www.facebook.com/painwithsex/

Stop the fear. Vaginismus: a painful spasmodic contraction of the vagina in response to physical contact or pressure, especially during sexual intercourse.

Vaginismus Support

https://www.facebook.com/groups/2358227762/ (Private group)

https://www.facebook.com/groups/Dyspareunia.Support/ (Private group)

This is a group where individuals suffering from vaginismus can discuss their experiences and support one another without judgment. Do not be embarrassed! Partners of individuals with vaginismus are also welcome!

Vaginismus, Vulvodynia, and Vulvar Vestibulitis Support Group

https://www.facebook.com/groups/872970066100928/ (Private group)

This is a support group for patients and supporters of Vaginismus, Vulvodynia, Vulvar Vestibulitis and related conditions. This group is open to people of any gender. This group is also open to health care providers if it is not used as a means for advertising. We will remove anyone who's intentions are questionable. This support group is intended as an avenue for us to share our experiences, frustrations, improvements, and achievements. This is a closed group; the posts will not show up in your newsfeed, but people will be able to see that you are a member of this group. It is the way Facebook is set up; unfortunately, there is no way around it.

Vestibulectomy Surgery and Vestibulodynia Support Group

https://www.facebook.com/groups/vestibulodynia.support (Private group)

This group is focused on helping women learn about Vestibulectomy Surgery for Vestibulodynia pain. We are here to support women through deciding to have the surgery, as well as support women through their recovery of surgery and thereafter. Vulvodynia is a generalized term for female genital pain, and Vestibulodynia is the term used more specifically to define pain in the vestibule. Vestibulectomy surgery has become a very successful option for women with provoked vestibulodynia, although some with minor unprovoked pain as well as mostly provoked pain do find it successful as well. Not all pain is created equal, not all experiences are the same. This surgery does not work for everyone, but the most important things is for the person considering surgery to be sure they are a candidate for the surgery, and make sure that they have a good surgeon with experience and good success rates.

This group is here for support, no one person knows all the answers, and no one person has all the questions; therefore, we are here to search, and discover those answers and questions together as a supportive group.

Vestibulite Vulvaire / Vestibulodynie

https://www.facebook.com/groups/54191626305/ (Private group)

Since vestibulitis is a sexual disease, we often keep it to ourselves and try to hide it from others. The purpose of this group is to promote awareness of this disease and to try to provide support and responses to women who have it. It is not necessary to be a woman suffering from this disease to join this group. I really hope that it reaches the greatest number of Internet users!

Vulva Warriors

https://www.facebook.com/groups/1006063052818424/ (Private group)

This group is for Women who are looking to learn how to heal holistically. We discuss unconventional healing methods including Herbs, Supplements, Urine Therapy, Turpentine, Colon Cleanses, Fasting and Medical Medium Protocol. We promote eating a diet mostly of whole plant foods. We encourage eating a plant-based diet with lots of fruit and vegetables These are the best medicine there is.

Yes, we are different, but we get results! This is a positive and encouraging place to support your healing journey and fully heal from Vulvodynia. We believe that everyone can heal this! Never give up!

Vulvar Vestibulitis Syndrome (VVS) & Vestibulodynia & Vulvodynia Awareness

https://www.facebook.com/groups/298606723605186/ (Private group)

This is a group is for anyone that suffers from vulvar vestibulitis, also known as vulvodynia or vestibulodynia. Vulvodynia, simply put, is chronic vulvar pain without an identifiable cause. The location, constancy, and severity of the pain vary among sufferers. Some women experience pain in only one area of the vulva, while others experience pain in multiple areas. The most reported symptom is burning, but women's descriptions of the pain vary. One woman reported her pain felt like "acid being poured on my skin," while another described it as "constant knife-like pain. We are hoping this very specific group can bring people who are suffering together to talk and support one another. Awareness needs to be spread and there needs to be hope and a cure!

Vulvodynia Awareness

https://www.facebook.com/awareness4vulvodynia/

Vulvodynia is a chronic vulva/vaginal pain condition. We share photos, quotes, info, etc. Submit your story via message & we will post it anonymously.

Vulvodynia Support

https://www.facebook.com/groups/2229472941/ (Private group)

Vulvodynia Support Group

https://www.facebook.com/groups/495451827671289/ (Private group)

I started this group for Women who are currently or have suffered from Vulvodynia, other types of Vulvar pain and/or Pelvic Floor Dysfunction. The purpose of this group is to be able to post questions, share information and support each other.

The Vulvodynia Support Group

https://www.facebook.com/groups/228845697160436/ (Private group)

We are a group of loving and kind friends supporting each other with our experience and knowledge. What makes this group so awesome are the genuinely caring members that are dealing with their own pain, yet give support, encouragement, compassion, inspiration, and hope, etc. Our hope is that people will find support here, share their experiences and coping mechanisms, connect with each other, and build friendships.

Young Vulvodynia Sufferers

https://www.facebook.com/groups/311234812887332/ (Private group)

This group is for those who suffer with Vulvodynia who: 1. Are below 35; 2. Have never been abused; 3. Have never had children or whose Vulvodynia started before those events, but preferably exclusive to those three rules. This group was made for us to be surrounded by peers who are more like us in medical background and life stage.

Vestibulite, vaginisme, vulvodynie, dyspareunie, endométriose

https://www.facebook.com/groups/580126912125260/ (Private group)

The purpose of this group is to help everyone who wants to learn about the subject. It is accessible to all. However, for those who would like to remain anonymous, a private group also exists, if you wish to be added, you just need to send a private message and the procedure to follow will be indicated to you. Testimonies are welcome. You can share your frustrations, your progress, your victories.

Google Groups

alt.support.inter-cystitis

https://groups.google.com/forum/?hl=en#!forum/alt.support.inter-cystitis

A newsgroup in which you will find posts from several vestibulodynia sufferers.

Instagram

@pelvicawarenessproject

https://www.instagram.com/pelvicawarenessproject/

Connection and education for women experiencing Pelvic Floor Dysfunction.

@pelvichealthguru

https://www.instagram.com/pelvichealthguru/

Peache, CA

Sharing my journey with Vulvodynia & Crohn's. Spreading awareness for pelvic pain and sober living. DM me for a copy of my free resource guide!

@pelvicpainproject

https://www.instagram.com/pelvicpainproject/

Hi, I'm Zoë! She/her support space for chronic pelvic pain. Formerly @vulvodyniaaccessproject

@the.happy.pelvis

https://www.instagram.com/the.happy.pelvis/

My journey through #chronicpain + raising awareness & supporting others around the #pfd #interstitialcystitis #endometriosis #fibromyalgia #lupus

@theunhappypelvis

https://www.instagram.com/theunhappypelvis/

Charlotte. Talking all things pain, chronic illness, lifestyle, mental health & more. Sharing real life stories on my blog: theunhappypelvis@gmail.com

@vaginismus_girl

https://www.instagram.com/vaginismus_girl/

Urvaginaisntbroken. Neither is mine! Let's laugh, get educated, and compare notes on all things pelvic floor dysfunction, vaginismus and vulvodynia diagnosed oct '19.

@vulvabrasil

https://www.instagram.com/vulvabrasil/

Support page for women suffering from sexual dysfunction.

#vaginism #vulvodynia #vulvodyniaawareness #dispareunia Breaking taboos

@vulvodyniastruggles

https://www.instagram.com/vulvodyniastruggles/

Sara, struggling with vulvodynia and painful days. Looking to give guidance. College student and aspiring teacher!

Podcasts

The Pelvic Health Podcast

https://podcasts.apple.com/us/podcast/the-pelvic-health-podcast/id1022705760?mt=2

Podcast for professionals, as well as the public, on all things related to pelvic health. Interviews with leading experts. Hosted by physiotherapist Lori Forner, BScH, MPhtySt, PhD candidate.

The Pelvic Messenger: Discussing Pelvic, Bladder, Bowel and Sexual Disorders

https://www.blogtalkradio.com/pelvicmessenger

Pelvic messenger, supported by the International Pelvic Pain Society and Beyond Basics Physical Therapy, is devoted to promoting diagnoses, recovery, and success in treating Chronic Pelvic Pain (CPP) conditions in men, women, and children. Furthermore, we are dedicated to improving patient and healthcare providers education on CPP. The managers, Amy Stein, DPT and Alexandra Milspaw, PhD want to accomplish this mission by discussing up to date topics and research on pelvic and sexual pain and dysfunction. Hosts: Alexandra Milspaw, PhD, Amy Stein, DPT, Alexandra Lange, DPT.

Mission Statement: To provide educational talk radio shows on various chronic pelvic pain topics. In addition, we seek to provide hope and healing to individuals who suffer from pain related symptoms.

We will be having shows on all the many diseases and syndromes, which can make up CPP. The show is a message of hope and healing. Stay posted to the International Pelvic Pain Society and Beyond Basics Physical Therapy blogs for bi-monthly guests and topics. We look forward to your calls and questions!

Pelvic Rehabilitation Medicine

Pelvic Rehabilitation Medicine at multiple locations

https://soundcloud.com/user-977535138

At Pelvic Rehabilitation Medicine, we treat whole human beings, not symptoms. In the body, everything is connected; and the pelvic region is the vital center of the body's connected functioning. Our physicians take an innovative approach, combining traditional medicine with holistic modalities and restorative and regenerative medicine. We treat both male and female patients who experience core muscle and nerve problems; chronic pelvic pain; and pelvic floor muscle dysfunction.

Pelvic Zen

Connected to Sullivan Physical Therapy, Austin, TX

https://www.blogtalkradio.com/pelviczen

Welcome to Pelvic Zen, a show designed to promote pelvic floor wellness in men and women. My name is Caitlin McCurdy-Robinson, and I will be the host of the show. I am a Physical Therapist at Sullivan Physical Therapy in Austin, TX. Our clinic specializes in women's and men's health conditions related to the pelvic floor. Examples of pelvic floor dysfunctions include urinary and fecal incontinence, prolapse, constipation, chronic pelvic pain, sexual pain and other sexual related issues, and prenatal/postpartum pain. While all these conditions are common, many people suffer in silence because they do not realize treatments are available or because they are embarrassed to discuss their symptoms with a healthcare professional. Whether you are experiencing symptoms and don't know what to do next or you are already seeking treatment for your symptoms, this show aims to provide information and resources that will be helpful to you in your recovery process.

PT Below the Waist

Connected to Sullivan Physical Therapy, Austin, TX

https://soundcloud.com/ptbelowthewaist

https://www.facebook.com/PTBelowTheWaistPodcast/

https://twitter.com/ptbelowthewaist

Jamille Niewiara and Jessica Chastka are co-hosts of their new podcast called "PT: Below the Waist," a patient-oriented podcast discussing topics related to pelvic floor physical therapy and how it addresses bladder, bowel, and sexual function issues. The podcast features two pelvic floor physical therapists casually conversing about their experiences and thoughts towards pelvic floor related issues. Every few weeks, they will be posting podcasts about different diagnoses, tips/recommendations to address symptoms, and interviews with medical professionals. Subscribe to their podcast on iTunes, follow them on Twitter @ PTBelowTheWaist, and like them on Facebook. Leave comments and questions on their email: PTBelowTheWaist@gmail.com. Sullivan Physical Therapy encourages you to listen to their podcasts and get enlightened about "Better Pee, Better Poo, Better Sex".

Twitter

ApprehensiveVagBlog (@BloggerElphieW)

https://twitter.com/BloggerElphieW

A blogger trying to cope with vaginismus, anxiety and sexual pain through humor and conversation.
http://theapprehensivevagina.wordpress.com

BlogAboutPelvicPain (@SaraKSauder)

https://twitter.com/SaraKSauder

A blog about pelvic pain.

blogaboutpelvicpain.com

BridgeforPelvicPain

@pelvicpainB4PP

https://twitter.com/pelvicpainB4PP

Our mission is to connect the global community of chronic pelvic and sexual pain patients to resources, education, and hope through an integrative approach.

The Happy Pelvis (@HappyPelvis)

Blogging my journey through #chronicpain + raising awareness and supporting others around the world #interstitialcystitis #endometriosis #pfd #fibromyalgia #lupus

thehappypelvis.ca

Pain Down There (@painfulsex)

https://twitter.com/painfulsex

We are a multidisciplinary team dedicated to healing chronic sexual, genital, and pelvic pain through education/instructional resources.

paindownthere.com

PelvicSanity (@NicoleCozeanDPT)

https://twitter.com/NicoleCozeanDPT

Nicole Cozean PT, DPT, WCS : Founder of PelvicSanity Pelvic Health
and Wellness : Author of The Interstitial Cystitis Solution : #GetPT1st
#pelvicpt #ChoosePT

pelvicsanity.com

Sarah For Hope (@WSHThereIsHope)

https://twitter.com/WSHThereIsHope

I suffer from painful sex and pelvic pain, and I have learned so much
through my journey which I want to share to provide hope for others.

WhenSexHurtsThereIsHope.com

Vaginismus Awareness (@vaginismus411)

https://twitter.com/vaginismus411

Information and discussion and support on Vaginismus for anyone
suffering. Cured by PT 2016 and cured hypertonic pelvic floor
dysfunction.

https://m.facebook.com/groups/2358227762 (Private group)

@vulvodyniasiren

https://twitter.com/vulvodyniasiren

Conversation about women's health including pelvic pain and related
surgery: #vulvodynia & #vestibulectomy

What is Vulvodynia (@VulvoAwareness)

https://twitter.com/VulvoAwareness

Spreading awareness on Vulvodynia. It is a condition that affects many
women of various backgrounds and ages.

Websites

Academy of Pelvic Health Physical Therapy

https://aptapelvichealth.org/

We are a community of physical therapy professionals changing the
conversation and perception about pelvic and abdominal health issues
worldwide.

The Happy Pelvis

https://thehappypelvis.ca/

I have lived with chronic pelvic pain most of my life but had my symptoms dismissed and misdiagnosed for over 15 years. Since 2018 I have been diagnosed with Interstitial Cystitis/BPS, Endometriosis, Pelvic Floor Dysfunction, Fibromyalgia and Lupus (SLE). I hopes that what I share on my blog will help others advocate for themselves, better navigate the healthcare system and find the care and treatment they deserve.

Interstitial Cystitis Network/IC Network

https://forum.ic-network.com/forum/related-conditions-to-interstitial-cystitis/ic-other-related-conditions/vulvodynia

Female IC patients often have vulvodynia problems. Discuss this here!

Pelvic Awareness Project

https://pelvicawarenessproject.org/

Since launching in 2016, the people behind the Pelvic Awareness Project have been working to meet our goal of helping more than one million women with pelvic floor disorders by 2025. To do this, we have collaborated with critical partners, including healthcare providers, educators, and organizations, each of whom brings unique value to our initiative to educate, treat, and provide pelvic health resources.

Vaginismus

https://www.vaginismus.com/

Vulvodynia Support

https://vulvodyniasupport.forumotion.net/

Does life feel like one huge pain in the Vulva? I have created this forum so that women living with Vulvodynia (Vulva Pain) can have a place to share, chat and support each other.

Yahoo Groups

The VulvarDisorders List Support Group

https://groups.yahoo.com/neo/groups/VulvarDisorders/info

An on-line support group for women who suffer from vulvar
vestibulitis, vulvodynia, lichen sclerosis, vaginitis, and other vulvar
disorders. Family members and medical professionals are welcome.

You Tube

Beyond Pelvic Pain

https://www.youtube.com/channel/UCpCZcxYZoswiQG61qU9xe4g/
videos

Hi there. My name is Mary Trevellyan. For over 25 years I suffered
from chronic pelvic pain that was caused from a highly difficult-to-
treat combination of endometriosis, interstitial cystitis and provoked
vestibulodynia. I know firsthand how the pain and suffering that pelvic
pain causes can touch every aspect of your life. I have also experienced
the immense blessings of becoming 100% pain free, which I have been
since 2012.

I learned the hard way how to get pain-free, so you don't have to. My
mission is to help women suffering from chronic pelvic pain, like you
or someone you love, avoid wasting time and money on unnecessary
mistakes and become pain-free far more quickly than I did.

Dagmar Khan

The site has videos on a variety of medical and psychological topics.
The relevant medical playlists are:

Vaginismus and Vulvodynia:
https://www.youtube.com/playlist?list=PLP3zQ7JEnl9oxVNqRDRX
nxA1loLFCRr0a

Pelvic Healing:
https://www.youtube.com/playlist?list=PLP3zQ7JEnl9qtls1bQJePh
OBmCWqskonv

Jill Osborne

National IC Support Group Leader, Interstitial Cystitis Network, https://www.ichelp.org/

https://www.youtube.com/channel/UCzFbz15quyoabP5_lL1i1Dg

Interstitial cystitis (IC), also known as painful bladder syndrome or bladder pain syndrome, affects millions of men and women throughout the world. Jill Heidi Osborne MA is the longest serving IC support group leader in the United States, having served for more than 25 years. Founder of the IC Network, Jill provides twice monthly live streamed support group meetings to help patients and their family members learn more about IC diagnosis, treatments, subtypes, flare management, diet and pain care. Jill has degrees in Chemistry, Pharmacology with a master's degree in psychology. The purpose of our support group meetings is to educate patients so that they can work more effectively with their medical care providers.

Series of videos entitled "Live IC and Pelvic Pain Support Group Meeting."

Meghin Uhl

Just a 26-year-old living with multiple chronic illnesses trying to live a normal life. I have a passion for beauty products, food, and going to bed at 9pm on a Friday night. Welcome to my life.

The site has medical and personal videos. The medical playlists are:

Vulvodynia and Pelvic Updates:
https://www.youtube.com/playlist?list=PLjADlQGAGcronyiOXdK7t r1dplRNSXDBn

Pelvic Floor Therapy:
https://www.youtube.com/playlist?list=PLjADlQGAGcrpAS6YCPff5 6SL6EDNgi1hF

Pelvic Dysfunction Explained:
https://www.youtube.com/playlist?list=PLjVdBniSq4ZQcKWHWcN AsKJF7OoORrnC1

Pelvic Pain Explained Webinar Series:
https://www.youtube.com/playlist?list=PLjVdBniSq4ZRZyb31LQ5T 8ofGUjCRHrov

PelvicSanity

https://www.youtube.com/channel/UCXigFK5hLLF82uZ72jzTvmg

PelvicSanity provides practical, positive information on pelvic pain
and dysfunction conditions.

From PelvicSanity physical therapy in Orange County, CA:
https://www.pelvicsanity.com/.

Roo Morgue

Hi! I'm Roo Morgue, a 24-year-old cam girl, altmodel and casual
writer from Manchester, UK. I occasionally upload with random
topics, mostly about my life.

The site has medical and personal videos. The medical playlists and
videos are:

Lichen Sclerosus and Vulvodynia:
https://www.youtube.com/playlist?list=PLFhMe7yxRDKnry6jo2Cs_
n8h6mzF68bVQ

Vulvodynia and Therapy: A rant:
https://www.youtube.com/watch?v=L1_QwHj3TtE

Karalee Vigstol

https://www.youtube.com/channel/UCw_KRW4LTX7nvIw9XKSbN
vA/

National Vulvodynia Association

https://www.youtube.com/c/NvaOrg/featured

The National Vulvodynia Association is a non-profit organization
committed to improving the health and quality of life of women
suffering with vulvodynia. To learn more please visit:
http://www.nva.org.

Vulvar Vernacular

https://www.youtube.com/channel/UC7mk-yzjB3Tfnk-G-l1nt7w

vulvarvernacular.wordpress.com

Vulvar Vernacular was created in 2015 to provide a network for women suffering from vulvar vestibulitis, vulvodynia, and similar chronic pain conditions. All content shared on this site is the opinion of the creator and should not be substituted for the opinions of medical professionals.

See also lists of local groups at:

The American Chronic Pain Association

https://www.theacpa.org/about-us/support-groups/

Interstitial Cystitis Association

https://www.ichelp.org/support/support-groups/us-support-groups/

https://www.inspire.com/groups/interstitial-cystitis-association/topic/support-groups/?origin=tfr (Online Support Community)

Interstitial Cystitis Network/IC Network

https://www.ic-network.com/ic-support-center/ic-support-groups/

https://forum.ic-network.com/forum/meet-others-by-region/interstitial-cystitis-support-group-list-usa-canada/31065-list-of-groups-by-state

International Pain Foundation

https://internationalpain.org/support-groups/

Chapter 30

Claiming Disability Benefits

The US Social Security Disability Benefits Program

The National Vulvodynia Association (NVA) explains that in America, the Social Security Administration (SSA) runs two different programs offering disability benefits.

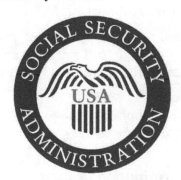

The first program is SSDI (Social Security Disability Insurance), which pays benefits to "insured" disabled people under 65 years old. (Note: those who are regarded as insured qualify according to the Social Security tax they have paid on their wages). In addition to this, the SSA may pay benefits to disabled dependents of insured individuals [1]. As with all regulations, these benefits are subject to change.

The second program is SSI (supplemental security income), which can be claimed by disabled people who have modest resources and income. Further, Medicare benefits are available to government employees who are "insured" and meet the Social Security Administration's definition of disability, and to those who have been eligible for SSDI for a period of 24 months [1].

Prepare Ahead of Time

As you get ready to apply for disability benefit, preparing everything in advance and making sure you have all the necessary information will help the process go smoothly. This way, your application will be up for processing right away, and you will receive your benefit sooner. A good way to prepare is to "List your treatment provider's information, your medications and work history for the past fifteen years and bring the document and medical records with you" [1].

How to Apply

When you formally apply for disability benefit, your medical assessments and records are not mandatory, but it may be helpful to provide them. If you do provide them, be sure to make copies. To apply, fill out a formal application for benefits, along with the Adult Disability and Work History Report [1].

You can find these resources and apply at www.ssa.gov/benefits/disability/. If you make an application online, print a copy before sending it, as you won't be able to make a copy once it is transmitted.

If you would like to apply over the phone or in person, call the administration staff at 800-772-1213 and they will give you an appointment [1].

Disability Determination Process

As soon as you complete your application, The SSA will pass on your forms to a state disability determination office, which will perform an initial disability determination and evaluation. The state office may ask for duplicates of your medical records from the offices where you were treated (as listed on your application). Next, the state office will work to determine what you may be entitled to, using the medical reports which you have given them or which they have received from your providers. Regardless of your reports, you may be asked to undertake an SSA-funded consultative examination [1].

Further Information

For more information, see "Benefits and Insurance for People with Disabilities" on the USA.gov website: www.usa.gov/disability-benefits-insurance. The site also has a live chat option.

The UK Disability Benefits

Disability Living Allowance for Adults

Adults who have a disability or suffer from long-term ill health can apply for a Personal Independence Payment, a new benefit which is slowly replacing DLA (Disabled Living Allowance). Note: if you are claiming a State Pension, then you should apply for Attendance Allowance instead [2].

Personal Independence Payment

PIP (Personal Independence Payment) is a tax-free benefit for individuals aged 16 and over, until they reach State Pension age. This payment is designed to help cover the extra expenses generated by a disability or long-term ill-health [2].

Attendance Allowance

Attendance Allowance is a tax-free benefit for individuals who are claiming a State Pension, suffering from a disability, and require someone to help look after them [2].

Employment and Support Allowance

If you are unable to work due to disability or illness, you might be able to get ESA (Employment and Support Allowance) [2].

Further Information

For more information, see the UK government website: https://www.gov.uk/financial-help-disabled/disability-and-sickness-benefits.

As with all regulations, benefits are subject to change.

Chapter 31

Basic Terminology

Acupuncture: a form of holistic medicine in which fine disposable needles are inserted in the skin, at points along what traditional Chinese medicine refers to as meridians (invisible lines of energy). It is used for the treatment of various physical and psychological conditions, including pain relief [1].

Anesthesia: pain relief through loss of sensation [2].

Anesthetics: pharmaceuticals that relieve pain [2].

Antidepressants: medications that are prescribed for the treatment of depression. They may be used for other purposes, including the treatment of neuropathic (nerve) pain, as in vulvodynia [2].

Biofeedback: a technique used by physical therapists to help patients control various body functions, such as unstable muscles in the pelvic walls [2].

Biopsy: a minor surgical procedure that involves removing a small piece of tissue from an area in the body such as the vulvar skin. This tissue is then examined under a laboratory microscope [2].

Cannabinoids: "naturally occurring compounds found in the Cannabis sativa plant. Of over 480 different compounds present in the plant, only around 66 are termed cannabinoids. The most well-known among these compounds is the delta-9-tetrahydrocannabinol (Δ9-THC), which is the main psychoactive ingredient in cannabis" [3].

Clitorodynia: an abnormal pain in the clitoris. Symptoms include a sharp, stabbing pain, irritation, or rawness, which can be aggravated by moving at certain angles, wearing tight underwear, walking, or touching. The most common cause of this condition is the buildup of a type of hard, sand grain-like material (known as keratin pearls), between the hood of the clitoris (prepuce), and the clitoris. Other drivers of clitorodynia that impact the vulva include various skin diseases such as lichen planus or lichen sclerosis, injury to the pudendal nerve or clitoral branch of the pudendal nerve, or a cyst or herniated disc in the lumbar or sacral spine [4].

Dyspareunia: persistent or recurrent genital pain that occurs just prior to, during, or after sexual intercourse. Symptoms vary and include only experiencing pain at sexual entry (penetration); feeling pain during every penetration, be it sexual or inserting a tampon into your vagina; aching or burning pain; experiencing deep pain during thrusting; or a throbbing pain which goes on for hours after sexual penetration [5]. Dyspareunia is classified as superficial and deep dyspareunia.

Estrogen: this female hormone is produced in the ovaries. Estrogen is essential for the development and growth of female secondary sexual characteristics such as breasts, armpit, and pubic hair; as well as the regulation of the reproductive system, and the menstrual cycle [2].

Genetic Disorders: disorders caused by a change in genes or chromosomes [2].

Gynecologist: a physician who specializes in women's health [2].

Hormone: a substance manufactured within the body by organs or cells. Hormones also control the function of organs or cells. A good example is the hormone estrogen, which regulates the function of female reproductive organs [2].

Inflammation: a localized physical condition involving pain, irritation, redness, and/or swelling of the body's tissues [2].

Neuropathic Pain: Pain caused by damage and/or dysfunction of parts of the nervous system. It generates a continual "burning pain with spontaneous sharp exacerbations and worsening from normal sensory triggers, causing considerable impact on the quality of life;

people must have experienced pain for at least three months, with a mean pain intensity greater than 3/10 on a pain scale" [4]. Generalized unprovoked vulvodynia meets this description [6].

Nociceptor: a type of receptor that senses pain [7].

Nociceptive Pain: refers to one of the two major categories of physical pain, with nociceptive pain being the most common. It is the result of potentially harmful stimuli being detected by nociceptors around the body [7].

Pelvic Floor: a layer of muscles that span the bottom of the pelvis and support the pelvic organs. Women's pelvic organs include the bowel, bladder, and uterus [2].

Radiofrequency: the use of radiofrequency waves for medical treatment [2]. Radiofrequency is a type of energy that combines electric and magnetic fields, and these fields radiate in waves.

Ultrasound: sound waves that can be used to investigate internal body structures, or to treat for certain conditions like vulvodynia [2].

Vestibulodynia: pain at the vestibule (entrance to the vagina). The vestibule includes glands that generate vaginal lubrication when a woman is sexually aroused. "For a woman with generalized vestibulodynia, the pain is constant. A woman with provoked vestibulodynia (PVD) has pain when the area is touched" [8].

Vestibule: the vaginal opening in the labia minora (the smaller inner folds of the vulva) [2].

Vestibulectomy: the surgical excision of painful tissue on the vaginal vestibule [2].

Vulva: the female external genital region [2].

Vulvodynia: long-lasting pain of the vulva which is not the result of a skin disease or infection. Vulvodynia is sometimes confused with other vulvovaginal issues, such as chronic spasm or tension in the muscles of the vulvar region [2].

Appendix A. Popular Oral Medications Which Can be Prescribed for Vulvodynia

Anticonvulsant Drugs Used to Treat Vulvodynia

Medicines used to inhibit epileptic seizures may also be used to control chronic pain syndromes, hence it may be used in vulvodynia. Anticonvulsant or Antiepileptic drugs (AEDs) need to start at a low dose then gradually be increased to minimize adverse effects and then tapered off if decided to discontinue treatment [10].

Carbamazepine

Generic Name: Carbamazepine (oral)

Brand Names: Tegretol XR, Tegretol, Equetro, Epitol, Carbatrol

Carbamazepine is classed as an anticonvulsant drug and works to decrease the nerve impulses which generate nerve pain and seizures [1].

Common Adverse Effects of Carbamazepine

Adverse effects may include: weakness, muscle aches, flu-like symptoms, swollen glands, fever, skin rash [1]. Some of the side effect are dose related and may be dose limiting.

When to Seek Immediate Help

Seek medical help immediately if you experience: an allergic reaction, unusual bruising, severe weakness, muscle ache, flu-like symptoms, swollen glands, a severe skin reaction, an allergic reaction, fever, yellowing of the eyes or skin, continuous back-and-forth eye movements or double or blurred vision [1].

Gabapentin

Generic Name: Gabapentin

Brand Names: Neurontin, Horizant, Gralise

Gabapentin is an anticonvulsant medication designed to target the nerves and chemicals linked to the cause of certain types of pain and seizures. All the gabapentin brands are given to adults for the treatment of nerve pain generated by various disorders. It is important to only take the form/brand of gabapentin that has been prescribed by your doctor [1].

Research Results

"In 3 out of 4 trials using oral gabapentin, the dosage was gradually increased based on tolerability and efficacy (benefit). Therefore, there are wide-ranging dosages, making it difficult to ascertain specific dose-response relationships. Three studies resulted in at least a partial response to therapy of roughly 60% to 80% of patients" [3].

Common Adverse Effects of Gabapentin

Adverse effects may include: changes in behavior; difficulties with memory; problems concentrating; acting in an aggressive, hostile, or restless way; tiredness, drowsiness, dizziness, headache; swelling in feet or hands; difficulty with your eyes; or problems with coordination [1].

When to Seek Immediate Help

Seek medical help immediately if you experience: an allergic reaction; swollen lymph nodes and/or fever, rash; severe tiredness or weakness; difficulties with muscle movement or balance; pain in the upper stomach; chest pain, trouble breathing, worsening or new cough with fever; severe numbness or tingling; rapid eye movement; kidney difficulties - no or little urination, difficult or painful urination, swelling in the ankles or feet [1].

Pregabalin

Generic Name: Pregabalin

Brand Name: Lyrica

Pregabalin is an anticonvulsant medication. It works to slow down impulses in the brain and impacts the brain chemicals which send pain signals throughout the nervous system. It helps reduce pain generated by various diseases [1].

Research Results

In one study on Pregabalin, it was noted that "42% of patients had between 80% and 100% relief of symptoms after progressing from TCA therapy failure" [3].

Common Adverse Effects of Pregabalin

Adverse effects may include: headache, fatigue, drowsiness, dizziness, constipation, weight gain, infection, loss of control of body movements, accidental injury, visual field loss, tremor, peripheral edema, double or blurred vision, or a dry mouth [1].

When to Seek Immediate Help

Seek medical help immediately if you experience: an allergic reaction, vision problems; tenderness, weakness, difficulty breathing; unusual bleeding, easy bruising, swelling in your feet or hands, dark colored urine, unusual lethargy, fever, unexplained muscle pain, or rapid weight gain (particularly if you have heart problems or diabetes) [1].

Levetiracetam

Generic Name: Levetiracetam

Brand Names: Spritam, Roweepra, Keppra XR, Keppra

Levetiracetam is another anticonvulsant medication that is used in the treatment of epilepsy, neuralgia, persistent headache, and bipolar disorder [1].

Common Adverse Effects of Levetiracetam

Adverse effects may include: infection, stuffy nose, loss of appetite, feeling irritable or aggressive; dizziness or drowsiness; tiredness or weakness [1].

When to Seek Immediate Help

Seek medical help immediately if you experience: an allergic reaction, a severe skin reaction, a mild or more serious rash, difficulties with movement or walking; feeling very tired or weak, extreme drowsiness, infection, weakness, a chill, fever, unusual bleeding; uncommon changes in mood or behavior, hallucinations, confusion, being irritable or talkative; easy bruising, loss of coordination or balance [1].

Lamotrigine

Generic Name: Lamotrigine

Brand Names: Lamictal XR, Lamictal ODT, Lamictal CD, Lamictal

Lamotrigine is an anticonvulsant drug, and although it is not regarded as an antidepressant, it is nonetheless, used to treat certain types of depression, and bipolar disorder [5].

Common Adverse Effects of Lamotrigine

Adverse effects may include: insomnia; tremor; fatigue or drowsiness; runny nose; sore throat; fever; headache; dizziness; blurred or double vision; dry mouth; nausea and vomiting; diarrhea; stomach pain; and gastrointestinal distress [5].

When to Seek Immediate Help

Seek medical help immediately if you experience: an allergic reaction such as a skin reaction; a rash; skin disorder; blistering or peeling skin; swollen glands; fever; sore throat; behavior or mood changes; greater sensitivity to light; headache; stiff neck; severe muscle pain; confusion; weakness; drowsiness; jaundice (yellowing of the eyes or skin); and burning painful sores in or around the genitals, eyes or mouth [5].

Oxcarbazepine

Generic Name: Oxcarbazepine

Brand Name: Trileptal, Oxtellar XR

Oxcarbazepine is another anticonvulsant drug which works to decrease the nerve impulses that generate pain [1]. Patients may need to be maintained on a specific brand.

Common Adverse Effects of Oxcarbazepine

Adverse effects may include, but are not limited to: a rash, double vision, shaking or tremors; vomiting, nausea, difficulties with coordination or balance, tiredness, drowsiness, or dizziness [1].

When to Seek Immediate Help

Seek medical help immediately if you experience: an allergic reaction, yellowing of your eyes or skin, fever, a skin rash, unusual bruising, severe weakness, muscle aches, flu-like symptoms, or swollen glands [1].

Electrolyte Imbalance

Oxcarbazepine can lower the body's sodium to low levels, and this can generate a life-threatening electrolyte imbalance. Symptoms include increased seizures, muscle pain, severe weakness, feeling irritable or tired, confusion, lack of energy, and nausea [1].

Topiramate

Generic Name: Topiramate

Brand Name: Topiragen, Trokendi XR, Topamax Sprinkle, Topamax, Qudexy XR Sprinkle

Topiramate is an anticonvulsant drug, which is also used to treat anxiety and depression, post-traumatic stress disorder, and bipolar disorder [1].

Common Adverse Effects of Topiramate

Adverse effects may include: allergic reaction, anorexia, mood changes, distorted sense of taste, weight loss, visual disturbance, depression, speech disturbance, psychomotor disturbance, pricking or tingling ('pins and needles') which are mainly generated by damage to/pressure on peripheral nerves; nervousness, nausea, memory impairment, poor concentration, fatigue, drowsiness, dizziness, diplopia (double vision), diarrhea, confusion, speech disorder, ataxia, and anxiety [1].

When to Seek Immediate Help

Seek medical help immediately if you experience: an allergic reaction, nervousness, confusion, problems with vision, as topiramate is associated with acute myopia with secondary angle-closure glaucoma - particularly rapidly decreasing vision, eye pain, double vision or blurred vision; tingling, prickling or burning sensations; unsteadiness or clumsiness; increased eye pressure, uncontrolled continuous rolling, or back-and-forth eye movements, eye redness; drowsiness, dizziness, general slowing down of physical and mental activity; problems paying attention or concentrating, memory difficulties; menstrual pain or changes; language or speech difficulties, or feeling unusually weak or tired [1].

Pregnancy and Contraception

A pregnancy test should be done before initiation of treatment as topiramate can cause major congenital malformations after exposure during the first trimester (the first twelve weeks of pregnancy) [12]. Fetal growth and prenatal monitoring are required.

Antidepressant Medications Used to Treat Vulvodynia

Antidepressants are grouped into classes based on their mode of action. These are selective serotonin reuptake inhibitors (SSRI's), serotonin-norepinephrine reuptake inhibitors (SNRI's), tricyclic antidepressants (TCA's), monoamine oxidase inhibitors (MAOI's) and atypical agents. Some of these classes and their drugs can be used for treatment and symptomatic relief of vulvodynia and are discussed below. This is not an extensive list.

Withdrawal and Stopping Antidepressants

When advised to stop treatment with an antidepressant drug, withdrawal effects may occur within 5 days of stopping. They are usually mild but, in some cases, may be significant. To reduce the effects of withdrawal symptoms, the dose should be reduced gradually over 4 weeks or longer, depending on how long the patient has been on treatment [7].

Suicidal Thoughts

When you first start taking an antidepressant medication, it's a good idea to monitor your mood, because a very small number of people, particularly those under the age of 24, can experience suicidal thoughts and behavior. It is important that you see your doctor regularly over the first 12 weeks of treatment (as a minimum) or if the dose has changed. This will allow you to tell your doctor about any new or worsening symptoms. These include "mood or behavior changes, anxiety, panic attacks, trouble sleeping, or if you feel impulsive, irritable, agitated, hostile, aggressive, restless, hyperactive (mentally or physically), feeling more depressed, or having thoughts about suicide or hurting yourself"[1]. Never suddenly stop taking antidepressants unless you have been directed to do so by your doctor, or you may experience unwelcome withdrawal symptoms. Your doctor will inform you how you can safely discontinue them [1].

Serotonin Syndrome

This is a rare but potentially serious adverse effect that is linked to certain antidepressants. Serotonin syndrome occurs when there are high levels of the chemical serotonin in the brain caused either by medication initiation, dose escalation, addition of new antidepressant, and replacing an antidepressant by another one without allowing a wash out period in between [6]. The adverse effects include tremor, rigidity, blood pressure changes, shivering, diarrhea, agitation, confusion, and muscle twitching. You should stop taking the medication under these circumstances and seek immediate advice from your doctor [6].

Tricyclic Antidepressants (TCA)

"Tricyclic antidepressants (the word tricyclic, refers to its chemical structure) have been the focus for both oral and topical therapies due to their dual effects in treating depression and neuropathic (nerve) pain. Amitriptyline has thus far been the most researched TCA and is widely used by healthcare professionals" [3]. Yet, due to the lack of a consistent method of assessing patients' pain, and the broad range of amitriptyline dosing, research into efficacy (benefit) is hindered [3].

There are certain contraindications (specific situations when a medication should not be used because it may be harmful) to taking TCAs and you should discuss with your doctor before commencing treatment. These can include:

- certain cardiac (heart) conditions
- certain mental health conditions
- certain diseases
- allergies
- interactions with other medicines

Common adverse effects of TCAs vary depending on the individual medicine. Common adverse effects include, but are not limited to:

- drowsiness/confusion
- palpitations
- tremor
- vision disturbances
- gastric disturbances (diarrhea and/or constipation)
- nausea and vomiting
- unusual taste
- mouth pain
- weight or appetite changes
- urinating less than normal
- rash or itching
- breast swelling
- difficulty having an orgasm
- decreased sex drive [1]

When to Seek Immediate Help

Seek medical help immediately if you experience any of the following:

- an allergic reaction
- an irregular or fast heartbeat
- the whites of your eyes turn yellow
- yellow skin
- frequent muscle cramps
- long-lasting weakness or confusion
- constant headaches
- eye pain
- swelling or redness in or around the eyes
- severe constipation
- being unable to pass urine
- intense abdominal pain
- thoughts about self-harm or suicide [4]

Amitriptyline

Generic Name: Amitriptyline

Brand Names: Endep, Elavil, Vanatrip, Tryptizol

Amitriptyline is a TCA used to treat patients who are suffering from depression and pain, working by modifying the brain chemicals serotonin and norepinephrine which may be imbalanced [1].

There are various contraindications to taking it, such as, but not limited to having recently suffered a heart attack; having certain mental health illnesses; diseases or allergies; if you are/or are planning to become pregnant, are breastfeeding; are going to have surgery; or if you are on/or have taken certain medications in recent weeks. These situations must be discussed with your doctor [1].

Common Adverse Effects of Amitriptyline

Adverse effects may include, but are not limited to: diarrhea, constipation, nausea, dry mouth, headache, upset stomach, irregular heartbeat, vomiting, nausea, unusual taste, mouth pain; weight or appetite changes; urinating less than normal; rash or itching; breast swelling; difficulty having an orgasm, decreased sex drive [1].

When to Seek Immediate Help

Seek medical help immediately if you experience: allergic reactions; unusual behavior or thoughts; a feeling of light-headedness as though you could faint; chest pain/pressure, pain spreading to your shoulder/jaw, sweating, nausea; fluttering/pounding heartbeats in your chest; hallucinations, confusion; a seizure (convulsion); difficult/painful urination; severe constipation; unusual bleeding or easy bruising; or suddenly feeling ill or weak, chills, fever, swollen/red gums, mouth sores, sore throat or trouble swallowing [1].

Dosulepin

Generic Name: Dosulepin

Brand Name: Prothiaden

Dosulepin is another tricyclic antidepressant. It works to elevate mood, and is used to treat major depressive disorder, generalized anxiety disorder, and nerve pain [4].

Common Adverse Effects of Dosulepin

Adverse effects may include: headache, dizziness, constipation, weakness, fatigue, sleepiness, dry mouth, trouble urinating [4].

When to Seek Immediate Help

Seek medical help immediately if you experience: an allergic reaction, an irregular or fast heartbeat; the whites of your eyes turn yellow; yellow skin, frequent muscle cramps, long-lasting weakness or confusion, constant headaches, eye pain, swelling or redness around or in the eyes; severe constipation, being unable to pass urine, resulting in intense stomach pain, thoughts about self-harm or suicide [4].

Nortriptyline

Generic Name: Nortriptyline

Brand Names: Aventyl HCl, Pamelor, Allegron

Nortriptyline is a TCA used to treat patients who are suffering from depression, by modifying the brain chemicals serotonin and norepinephrine which may be imbalanced [1]. In addition, it is used to treat nerve pain (neuropathic) pain.

Common Adverse Effects of Nortriptyline

Adverse effects may include but are not limited to: changes in vision; constipation, loss of appetite, vomiting, nausea; anxiety, insomnia; dry mouth, unusual taste; swelling in the breast; trouble reaching orgasm, decreased sex drive [1].

When to Seek Immediate Help

Seek medical help immediately if you experience: allergic reactions; see halos around lights, swelling or eye pain; tunnel vision or blurred vision; restless muscle movements in your neck, jaw or tongue; a feeling of light-headedness as though you might faint; convulsions; worsening or new chest pain, fluttering in the chest or pounding heartbeats; sudden weakness or numbness; difficulty with balance, speech or vision; unusual bleeding, easy bruising, sore throat or fever; yellowing of the eyes or skin; difficult or painful urination; high serotonin levels- fainting, loss of coordination, diarrhea, vomiting, nausea, agitation, overactive reflexes, fast heart rate, fever, hallucinations [1].

Selective Serotonin and Norepinephrine Reuptake Inhibitor Antidepressants (SSNRI)

The mode of action of this class of drugs works differently than TCA's. These medications may be used to treat depression and anxiety disorders, as well as widespread body pain and peripheral neuropathy. The drugs used to treat vulvodynia include duloxetine and venlafaxine [10,11].

Duloxetine

Generic Name: Duloxetine

Brand Names: Irenka (US brand), Cymbalta (UK brand)

Duloxetine is an SSNRI used to treat patients who are suffering from major depression disorders and general anxiety. It works by modifying the brain chemicals serotonin and norepinephrine which may be imbalanced. In addition to this, it is used to treat chronic nerve pain and fibromyalgia [1].

Common Adverse Effects of Duloxetine

Adverse effects may include: increased sweating, dry mouth, loss of appetite, constipation, nausea, or drowsiness [1].

When to Seek Immediate Help

Seek medical help immediately if you experience: an allergic reaction or a severe skin reaction. Or if you experience any symptoms of serotonin syndrome, including diarrhea, vomiting, nausea, loss of coordination, twitching, muscle stiffness, fast heart rate, shivering, sweating, fever, hallucinations, or agitation [1].

Venlafaxine

Generic Name: Venlafaxine

Brand Names: Effexor, Effexor XL

Venlafaxine is an SSNRI used to treat patients who are suffering from panic disorder, anxiety, and major depressive disorder, by modifying the brain chemicals serotonin and norepinephrine which may be imbalanced [1]. It is also used in the treatment of nerve (neuropathic) pain.

Common Adverse Effects of Venlafaxine

Adverse effects may include: dry mouth, excessive sweating, delayed ejaculation, reduced appetite, anorexia, headache, nervousness, nausea, difficulty sleeping, drowsiness, dizziness, constipation, physical weakness, lack of energy, or difficulty reaching orgasm [1].

When to Seek Immediate Help

Seek medical help immediately if you experience: allergic reactions, see halos around lights, eye swelling or pain, tunnel or blurred vision, bleeding gums or nose, bleed or bruise easily, blood in stools or urine, cough up blood; difficulty breathing, tight chest, cough; convulsions; low sodium levels - slow breathing, feeling unsteady, hallucinations, vomiting, severe weakness, slurred speech, confusion or headache; symptoms of serotonin syndrome - fainting, loss of coordination, diarrhea, vomiting, nausea, agitation, overactive reflexes, fast heart rate, fever, hallucinations; severe nervous system reaction - tremors, uneven heartbeat, rigid muscles, confusion, sweating, high fever, feeling as though you might faint [1].

Selective Serotonin Reuptake Inhibitor (SSRI) Antidepressants

The medications in this class are generally tolerated well as they are less sedating and have fewer adverse effects. But they are poor in treating nerve (neuropathic) pain. They are considered a second option either alone or in combination with an anticonvulsant or if the patient is not tolerating TCA's [3].

Paroxetine

Generic Name: Paroxetine

Brand Names: Pexev, Paxil CR, Paxil, Brisdelle, Seroxat

Paroxetine is an SSRI (selective serotonin reuptake inhibitor) medication. It works to modify the brain chemical serotonin more than norepinephrine which may be unbalanced in patients who suffer from anxiety, depression, or other disorders. It is used to treat anxiety disorders; depression, and major depressive disorder, obsessive-compulsive disorder, and panic disorder [1].

Common Adverse Effects of Paroxetine

Adverse effects may include: an allergic reaction; a dry mouth; sweating; delayed ejaculation; decreased libido; headache; nausea;

insomnia; drowsiness; dizziness; diarrhea; constipation; and tiredness [1].

When to Seek Immediate Help

Seek medical help immediately if you experience: an allergic reaction; symptoms of serotonin syndrome, including loss of coordination, twitching, muscle stiffness, rapid heart rate, nausea, shivering, sweating, fever, agitation, hallucinations, diarrhea, or vomiting. Or a loss of coordination, feeling unsteady, slurred speech, severe weakness, confusion, or headache brought about by low sodium levels in the body; a severe nervous reaction including fainting, tremors, uneven or fast heartbeats, confusion, sweating, high fever, or extremely stiff muscles; coughing up blood; or unusual bleeding in the rectum, vagina, mouth, or nose; changes in appetite or weight; unusual tenderness or bone pain; bruising or swelling; seeing halos around lights, eye swelling or pain, tunnel vision, or blurred vision; feelings of extreme sadness or happiness; or unusual risk-taking behavior [1].

Benzodiazepines used to Treat Vulvodynia

Benzodiazepines are a category of psychoactive medications, which are used for treating several conditions including anxiety. They can trigger a tranquillizing chemical within the brain thereby increasing the risk of sedation. Patients need to be monitored for signs of respiratory depression and should also avoid if possible, co-prescribing benzodiazepines and opioids together, to avoid additive CNS depressant effects [13]. Benzodiazepines should only be used for a short period of time. Avoid abrupt withdrawal. Benzodiazepines also have paradoxical effects such as increased aggression and ranges from talkativeness, excitement, and antisocial acts [13].

Clonazepam

Generic Name: Clonazepam

Brand Names: KlonoPIN, Rivotril

Clonazepam works by modifying unbalanced brain chemicals, to ameliorate various forms of anxiety disorder [1].

Common Adverse Effects of Clonazepam

Adverse effects may include: cough, sore gums, elevated saliva production, weight change, change in sexual desire, excessive hair loss or growth, muscle pain, blurred vision, dizziness, or drowsiness [1]. Some of these side effects are similar in all benzodiazepines.

When to Seek Immediate Help

Seek medical help immediately if you experience: an allergic reaction, involuntary or unusual eye movements, fluttering or pounding heartbeats in the chest; shallow or weak breathing; thoughts of self-harming or suicide; unusual changes in behavior or mood; hallucinations, aggression, confusion, or severe drowsiness [1].

Opioids Used to Treat Vulvodynia

Opioids including tramadol and tapentadol (weak opioids); oxycodone and morphine (strong opioids) may be used in short-term use during a vulvodynia pain flare-up, to relieve pain. They can also be used in initial treatment while you gradually increase the dose of an anticonvulsant or antidepressant to a therapeutic level [10].

Tapentadol

Generic Name: Tapentadol

Brand Names: Nucynta ER, Nucynta (USA available brand), Palexia, Palexia SR (UK available brand)

Tapentadol is as an opioid pain medication (narcotic). It is used to treat patients who suffer moderate to severe pain [1]. There is a risk of seizures with tapentadol and should be used in cautions with patients with a history of seizure disorders, patients taking anti-depressants and anti-psychotics.

Common Adverse Effects of Tapentadol

Adverse effects may include but are not limited to: anxiety, decreased appetite, body temperature change, muscle spasms, vomiting; nausea; drowsiness; dry mouth; severe itching skin; and constipation [1]. Other adverse effects that are common to other opioids include respiratory depression, dependence, confusion, dizziness, flushing, headache, hallucinations.

When to Seek Immediate Help

Seek medical help immediately if you experience: an allergic reaction; blue colored lips; slow breathing, especially with long pauses; stopping breathing during sleep; shallow breathing; feeling light-headed as though you are going to faint; feeling hot; being agitated; convulsion; confusion; severe dizziness or drowsiness; trouble with balance or speech. Or serotonin syndrome, which includes nausea; loss of coordination; twitching; muscle stiffness; rapid heart rate; shivering; sweating; fever; hallucinations; agitation; diarrhea or vomiting [1].

Tramadol

Generic Name: Tramadol

Brand Names: Ultram ER, Ultram, ConZip, Zydol

Tramadol is a narcotic-like pain reliever which also increases norepinephrine levels in nerves. It is prescribed to patients who suffer from moderate to severe pain [1].

Common Adverse Effects of Tramadol

Adverse effects may include: headache; tiredness; feeling drowsy; dizziness; stomach pain; vomiting; nausea or constipation [1].

When to Seek Immediate Help

Seek medical help immediately if you experience: stopping breathing while sleeping; shallow breathing; sighing; noisy breathing; a weak pulse or slow heart rate; feeling light-headed as though you might faint; convulsion; feeling more weak or tired; dizziness; vomiting; loss of appetite. Or serotonin syndrome symptoms, including diarrhea; vomiting; nausea; loss of coordination; twitching; muscle stiffness; fast heart rate; shivering; sweating; fever; hallucinations; or agitation [1]

Appendix B. References

Understanding Vulvodynia
and Getting a Diagnosis

Chapter 1. What is Vulvodynia?

[1]. Hinde, Natasha (2019). "Vulvodynia: Symptoms and Treatment Explained." https://www.huffingtonpost.co.uk/entry/vulvodynia-symptoms-and-treatment_uk_59b7ae19e4b027c149e2216d?guccounter=1&guce_referrer=aHR0cHM6Ly93d3cuZ29vZ2xlLmNvbS8&guce_referrer_sig=AQAAAM0_pWiIHJ8gHsv--LmXoqPTK1Nl6iSDHGIoWnGseV6PHnoJDwDVLsxl4sdf21uRDfgxoxybUsuXv2ZyKCDaDaEH996fzsEGSfnATozt8Hqkgc1UpCmvKlyhDjlMze8BKZq2RZzWqvGy2wGK-caz3tLK7veYiPb4dZsTHnzp1VA-

[2]. Chalmers et al. (2016). "The role of physiotherapy in the management of vulvodynia." https://www.bodyinmind.org/wp-content/uploads/Chalmers-et-al-2016-The-physiotherapy-management-of-vulvodynia.pdf

[3]. Nagandla, G. & Sivalingam, N. (2014). "Vulvodynia: integrating current knowledge into clinical practice." Obstetrics & Gynaecology. https://obgyn.onlinelibrary.wiley.com/doi/full/10.1111/tog.12130

[4]. Scott, Trudy (2019). "Vulvodynia: oxalates, GABA, tryptophan and physical therapy." Every Woman Over 29. https://www.everywomanover29.com/blog/vulvodynia-oxalates-gaba-tryptophan-physical-therapy/

[5]. National Vulvodynia Association (2019). https://www.nva.org/what-is-vulvodynia/

[6]. National Vulvodynia Association (2019). "Vulvodynia: Get the Facts." https://www.nva.org/media-center/

[7]. Harvard health Publishing (2019). "By the way, doctor: What can I do about vulvodynia?" https://www.health.harvard.edu/newsletter_article/what-can-i-do-about-vulvodynia

[8]. Graziottin, Alessandra, Murina, Filippo (2011). Clinical Management of Vulvodynia. Milan: Springer.

[9]. Glazer, H.I; Rodke, G. (2002). The Vulvodynia Survival Guide. California: Harbinger Publications.

[10]. Mount Sinai (2019). "Vulvodynia." https://www.mountsinai.org/health-library/diseases-conditions/vulvodynia

[11]. Amherd, Claudia (2014). Freeing Yourself From Pelvic Pain. Self-Published.

[12]. Dunkley, C.R; Brotto, L.A. (2016). Psychological Treatments for Provoked Vestibulodynia: Integration of Mindfulness-Based and Cognitive Behavioral Therapies. Journal of Clinical Psychology. https://www.researchgate.net/publication/299475036_Psychological_Treatmen

ts_for_Provoked_Vestibulodynia_Integration_of_Mindfulness-Based_and_Cognitive_Behavioral_Therapies/link/5ccb0a2e92851c3c2f81677f/download

[13]. NIH (2019). "Randomized CO2 vs Sham Laser Treatment of Provoked Vestibulodynia." https://clinicaltrials.gov/ct2/show/NCT03390049

[14]. Judge, D.E. (2002). "What You Can Do About Vulvar Pain." NEJM Journal Watch. https://www.jwatch.org/wh200201080000014/2002/01/08/what-you-can-do-about-vulvar-pain

[15]. National Vulvodynia Association (N.d.). "Vulvodynia: A Self-Help Guide." http://www.isswsh.org/images/PDF/NVA.Self-help.guide.pdf

[16]. Meijden et al,. (2016). "2016 European guideline for the management of vulval conditions." https://www.iusti.org/regions/europe/pdf/2017/Vulvalconditions.pdf

Chapter 2. Understanding the Basics

[1]. National Vulvodynia Association (N.d.). "Vulvodynia: A Self-Help Guide." http://www.isswsh.org/images/PDF/NVA.Self-help.guide.pdf

Chapter 3. Getting a Diagnosis

[1]. NIH (2017). "How do health care providers diagnose vulvodynia?" https://www.nichd.nih.gov/health/topics/vulvodynia/conditioninfo/diagnosed

[2]. Chalmers et al. (2016). "The role of physiotherapy in the management of vulvodynia." https://www.bodyinmind.org/wp-content/uploads/Chalmers-et-al-2016-The-physiotherapy-management-of-vulvodynia.pdf

[3]. Mayo Clinic (2017). "Vulvodynia." https://www.mayoclinic.org/diseases-conditions/vulvodynia/diagnosis-treatment/drc-20353427

[4]. Nagandla, G. & Sivalingam, N. (2014). "Vulvodynia: integrating current knowledge into clinical practice." Obstetrics & Gynecology. https://obgyn.onlinelibrary.wiley.com/doi/full/10.1111/tog.12130

[5]. Harvard Health Publishing (2019). "By the way, doctor: What can I do about vulvodynia?" https://www.health.harvard.edu/newsletter_article/what-can-i-do-about-vulvodynia

[6]. National Vulvodynia Association (2019). "Vulvodynia: Get the Facts." https://www.nva.org/media-center/

[7]. Bhide AA, Puccini F, Bray R, Khullar V, Digesu GA. (2015). "The pelvic floor muscle hyperalgesia (PFMH) scoring system: a new classification tool to assess women with chronic pelvic pain: multicentre pilot study of validity and reliability." Eur J Obstet Gynecol Reprod Biol. 2015 Oct;193:111-3. doi: 10.1016/j.ejogrb.2015.07.008. Epub 2015 Jul 31.

[8]. Taylor – Robinson D. Horner P. & Pallecaros A. (2020) "Understanding the terms we use: support for using 'sexually shared microbiota' (SSM)" International Journal of STD & AIDs https://pubmed.ncbi.nlm.nih.gov/31948339/

Chapter 4. Vulva Self-Help Tips

[1]. Cleveland Clinic (2019). "Vulvar Care."
https://my.clevelandclinic.org/health/articles/4976-vulvar-care

[2]. UI Hospitals & Clinics (2018). "Vulvar skin care guidelines."
https://uihc.org/health-topics/vulvar-skin-care-guidelines

[3]. Ottawa Hospital. "Vulva Care."
https://www.ottawahospital.on.ca/en/documents/2017/01/vulvar-care-e.pdf/

Chapter 5. Five Things Anyone with a Vagina Needs to Know

[1]. McGrath, Paula (2019). "Five things everyone with a vagina should know." BBC
https://www.bbc.co.uk/news/health-50289607

[2]. Healthline (2019). "How to Clean Your Vagina and Vulva."
https://www.healthline.com/health/how-to-clean-your-vagina

Treatments for Vulvodynia

Chapter 6. Summary of Treatment Options for Vulvodynia

[1]. De Andres J, Sanchis-Lopez N, Asensio-Samper JM, Fabregat-Cid G, Villanueva-Perez VL, Monsalve Dolz V, Minguez A. (2016). "Vulvodynia--An Evidence-Based Literature Review and Proposed Treatment Algorithm." *Pain Pract.* 2016 Feb; 16(2):204-36.

Chapter 7. Oral Medication for Vulvodynia

See Appendix A. Popular Oral Medications Which Can be Prescribed for Vulvodynia

Chapter 8. Topical Medication for Vulvodynia

[1]. Boardman LA, Cooper AS, Blais LR, Raker CA. Topical gabapentin in the treatment of localized and generalized vulvodynia. Obstet Gynecol. 2008;112(3):579-85.

[2]. Foster DC, Kotok MB, Huang LS, et al. Oral desipramine and topical lidocaine for vulvodynia: a randomized controlled trial. Obstet Gynecol. 2010;116(3):583-93.

[3]. N Attal, Pharmacological Treatments of Neuropathic Pain: The Latest Recommendations. Rev Neurol (Paris). Jan-Feb 2019;175(1-2):46-50.

[4]. Harmer JP, Larson BS. Pain Relief from Baclofen Analgesia in a Neuropathic Pain Patient Who Failed Opioid and Pharmacotherapy: Case Report. J Pain Palliat Care Pharmacother. 2002;16(3):61-4.

[5]. Keppel Hesselink JM, Kopsky DJ, Sajben NL. Vulvodynia and proctodynia treated with topical baclofen 5 % and palmitoylethanolamide. Arch Gynecol Obstet. 2014;290(2):389-93.

[6]. Steinberg AC, Oyama IA, Rejba AE, Kellogg-Spadt S, Whitmore KE. Capsaicin for the Treatment of Vulvar Vestibulitis. Am J Obstet Gynecol. 2005 May;192(5):1549-53.

[7.] Vasileva, Polina; Strashilov, Strahil A.; Yordanov, Angel D. Aetiology, diagnosis, and clinical management of vulvodynia. Source: Menopausal Review / Przeglad Menopauzalny. 2020, Vol. 19 Issue 1, p44-48. 5p.

Chapter 9. Medical Cannabis for Vulvodynia

[1]. Grinspoon, P. (2019). "Cannabidiol (CBD) — what we know and what we don't." https://www.health.harvard.edu/blog/cannabidiol-cbd-what-we-know-and-what-we-dont-2018082414476

[2]. Moore, Genevieve R. (2019). "Cannabinoids & Your Vagina: the Science of Pleasure & Relief." Foria Wellness. https://www.foriawellness.com/blogs/learn/cbd-thc-vagina-sex-pleasure-relief

[3]. Fontaine, M. (2018). "Using Cannabis to Treat Persistent Pelvic Pain." https://pelvicpainrehab.com/pelvic-health/5726/using-cannabis-to-treat-persistent-pelvic-pain/

[4]. Doward, J. (2019). "Medical cannabis: Why are doctors still not prescribing it?" https://www.theguardian.com/society/2019/nov/03/medical-cannabis-patients-refused-drug-nhs-legalised

[5]. Wilson, D.R. (2019) "CBD vs. THC: What's the Difference" Healthline. [Online]. Available at: https://www.healthline.com/health/cbd-vs-thc [Accessed 27 June 2020]

[6]. Capano.A., Weaver. R. and Burkman. E. (2019). "Evaluation of the effects of CBD hemp extract on opioid use and quality of life indicators in chronic pain patients: a prospective cohort study." Postgraduate Medicine, 132 (1), pp. 56-61.

[7]. Van de Donk. T., Niesters. M., Kowal. M.A., Olofsen. E., Dahan. A. and Van Velzen. M. (2019). "An Experimental Randomized Study on The Analgesic Effects of Pharmaceutical-grade Cannabis in Chronic Pain Patients with Fibromyalgia." The Journal of International Association for the Study of Pain, 160 (4), pp. 860-869.

Chapter 10. Pelvic Floor Muscles and Physiotherapy for Vulvodynia

[1]. UChicago Medicine (2020). "Pelvic Floor Disorders". https://www.uchicagomedicine.org/conditions-services/pelvic-health/pelvic-floor-disorders

[2]. Berghmans, B. "Physiotherapy for pelvic pain and female sexual dysfunction: an untapped resource", Int Urogynecol J. 2018; 29(5): 631–638. https://www.ncbi.nlm.nih.gov/pmc/articles/PMC5913379/

[3]. Kegel 8 (2020). "What is the Pelvic Floor?"
https://www.kegel8.co.uk/advice/pelvic-floor-exercise/what-is-the-pelvic-floor.html

[4]. Hilde et al. "Postpartum Pelvic Floor Muscle Training and Urinary Incontinence".
Obstet Gynecol 2013 Dec;122(6):1231-8.
https://pubmed.ncbi.nlm.nih.gov/24201679/

[5]. "Pelvic Health Solutions: Educating health care professionals about pelvic health
since 2010" (2020).
https://pelvichealthsolutions.ca/for-the-patient/what-is-pelvic-floor-physiotherapy/

[6]. Wallace et al. (2019). "Pelvic floor physical therapy in the treatment of pelvic floor
dysfunction in women."
https://urology.stanford.edu/content/dam/sm/urology/JJimages/publications/
Pelvic-floor-physical-therapy-in-the-treatment-of-pelvic-floor-dysfunction-in-
women.pdf

[7]. Prendergast, Stephanie (2017). "Pelvic floor physical therapy for vulvodynia: a
clinician's guide." https://pelvicpainrehab.com/female-pelvic-pain/4354/pelvic-
floor-physical-therapy-vulvodynia/

[8]. Stein, Amy & Sauder, Sara. K (2017). "On the Backs of Giants: The Evolution of
Biofeedback in the Treatment of Vulvodynia." The Journal of Sexual Medicine.
2017; 14:1e2. https://www.jsm.jsexmed.org/article/S1743-6095(16)30816-5/pdf
oop;['/]#]#

[9]. Amy, Shirley (2015). The Winning Way to Quit Smoking. USA: Createspace.
https://www.amazon.com/Winning-Way-Quit-Smoking-ebook-dp-
B007QYD98S/dp/B007QYD98S/ref=mt_kindle?_encoding=UTF8&me=&qid=1
365674793

[10]. Bo et al. "An International Urogynecological Association (IUGA)/ International
Continence Society (ICS) joint report on the terminology for the conservative and
nonpharmacological management of female pelvic floor dysfunction". Int
Urogynecol J (2017) 28:191–213.
file:///C:/Users/User/Desktop/Bo%20et%20al%202017.pdf

[11]. Rogers et al. "An International Urogynecological Association
(IUGA)/International Continence Society (ICS) joint report on the terminology
for the assessment of sexual health of women with pelvic floor dysfunction".
Neurourol Urodyn. 2018;37(4):1220-1240.

Chapter 11. Biofeedback for Vulvodynia

[1]. Women's Health Matters (2020). "Treatment."
https://www.womenshealthmatters.ca/health-centres/pelvic-
health/vulvodynia/treatment/

[2]. Stanton, A.M., Kirakosian, N. "The Role of Biofeedback in the Treatment of Sexual
Dysfunction". Curr Sex Health Rep 12, 49–55 (2020).
https://link.springer.com/article/10.1007/s11930-020-00257-5

[3]. The Mayo Clinic. "Biofeedback." https://www.mayoclinic.org/tests-
procedures/biofeedback/about/pac-20384664

[4]. Rao SS. "Dyssynergic defecation and biofeedback therapy". Gastroenterol Clin North Am. 2008;37(3):569-viii. doi:10.1016/j.gtc.2008.06.011 http://www.ncbi.nlm.nih.gov/pmc/articles/PMC2575098/

[5]. Van Ark, A. 9(2010). "What is Biofeedback?" http://www.vabs.nl/biofeedback/wat-is-biofeedback

[6]. Stein, Amy & Sauder, Sara. K (2017). "On the Backs of Giants: The Evolution of Biofeedback in the Treatment of Vulvodynia." The Journal of Sexual Medicine. 2017;14:1e2. https://www.jsm.jsexmed.org/article/S1743-6095(16)30816-5/pdf

[7]. Physiopedia (2020). "Biofeedback".https://www.physio-pedia.com/Biofeedback#cite_note-3

[8]. Berghmans, B. "Physiotherapy for pelvic pain and female sexual dysfunction: an untapped resource", Int Urogynecol J. 2018; 29(5): 631–638.

Chapter 12. Desensitization using Dilators and Vibrators for Vulvodynia

[1]. Berghmans, B. "Physiotherapy for pelvic pain and female sexual dysfunction: an untapped resource", Int Urogynecol J. 2018; 29(5): 631–638. https://www.ncbi.nlm.nih.gov/pmc/articles/PMC5913379/

[2]. The Vulva Pain Society (2019). "Physiotherapy." http://vulvalpainsociety.org/vps/index.php/treatments/physiotherapy

[3]. Prendergast, Stephanie (2017). "Pelvic floor physical therapy for vulvodynia: a clinician's guide." https://pelvicpainrehab.com/female-pelvic-pain/4354/pelvic-floor-physical-therapy-vulvodynia/

[4]. The Vulvar Pain Society (2019). "Physiotherapy." http://vulvalpainsociety.org/vps/index.php/treatments/physiotherapy

Chapter 13. Pelvic Floor Training Chairs for Vulvodynia

[1]. Cosmetech UK (2018). "The Pelvic Training Chair." https://www.cosmetech.co.uk/wp-content/uploads/2018/01/Pelvic-Floor-Brochure.pdf

[2]. Lim R, Liong ML, Leong WS, Karim Khan NA, Yuen KH. Pulsed Magnetic Stimulation for Stress Urinary Incontinence: 1-Year Followup Results. J Urol. 2017;197(5):1302-1308. https://pubmed.ncbi.nlm.nih.gov/27871927/

[3]. "BTL-6000 Super Inductive System Locus Clinical Evidence." (2020). https://theurologypartnership.co.uk/wp-content/uploads/2020/10/btl-emsella-chair-clinical-evidence.pdf

Chapter 14. Can a Nerve Block Help Relieve Vulvodynia?

[1]. Mayo Clinic (2017). "Vulvodynia." https://www.mayoclinic.org/diseases-conditions/vulvodynia/diagnosis-treatment/drc-20353427

[2]. The London Pain Clinic (2020). "Pudendal Nerve Blocks for the Treatment of Vulvodynia." https://www.londonpainclinic.com/antineuropathic-medication/pudendal-nerve-blocks-for-the-treatment-of-vulvodynia/

[3]. UR Medicine (2020). "Pudendal Nerve Block." https://www.urmc.rochester.edu/imaging/patients/procedures/pudendal-block.aspx

[4]. London Pain Clinic (2020.). "Pudendal Nerve Pulsed Radiofrequency (PRF) for the Treatment of Vulvodynia." https://www.londonpainclinic.com/minimally-invasive-pain-management/pudendal-nerve-pulsed-radiofrequency-prf-for-the-treatment-of-vulvodynia/

[5]. De Seta, Francesco & Raichi, Mauro (2018). "Dynamic quadripolar RadioFrequency and vulvodynia." University of Milan. Oat. https://www.oatext.com/dynamic-quadripolar-radiofrequency-and-vulvodynia.php#Article

Chapter 15. How Botulinum Toxin (Botox®/Dysport®) Can Help Vulvodynia

[1]. Yoon et al. "Botulinum toxin A for the management of vulvodynia." International Journal of Impotence Research, 2007 Jan-Feb;19(1):84-7 https://www.nature.com/articles/3901487

[2]. Falsetta et al. (2016). "A review of the available clinical therapies for vulvodynia management and new data implicating proinflammatory mediators in pain elicitation." BJOG. https://obgyn.onlinelibrary.wiley.com/doi/pdf/10.1111/1471-0528.14157

[3]. Petersen CD, Giraldi A, Lundvall L, Kristensen E. Botulinum toxin type A-a novel treatment for provoked vestibulodynia? Results from a randomized, placebo controlled, double blinded study. J Sex Med. 2009;6(9):2523-2537. https://pubmed.ncbi.nlm.nih.gov/19619148/

[4]. Diomande I, Gabriel N, Kashiwagi M, et al. Subcutaneous botulinum toxin type A injections for provoked vestibulodynia: a randomized placebo-controlled trial and exploratory subanalysis. Arch Gynecol Obstet. 2019;299(4):993-1000. https://pubmed.ncbi.nlm.nih.gov/30707361/

[5]. Pelletier F, Parratte B, Penz S et al. "Efficacy of high doses of botulinum toxin A for treating provoked vestibulodynia." B J of Dermatology 2011; 164 : 617-622. https://www.ipm.org.uk/15/news-archive/post/2/efficacy-of-high-doses-of-botulinum-toxin-a-for-treating-provoked-vestibulodynia

[6]. Pelletier F, Girardin M, Humbert P, Puyraveau M, Aubin F, Parratte B. Long-term assessment of effectiveness and quality of life of OnabotulinumtoxinA injections in provoked vestibulodynia. J Eur Acad Dermatol Venereol. 2016;30(1):106-111. https://pubmed.ncbi.nlm.nih.gov/26491951/

[7.] Jeon Y, Kim Y, Shim B, Yoon H, Park Y, Shim B, Jeong W, Lee D. A retrospective study of the management of vulvodynia. Korean J Urol. 2013 Jan;54(1):48-52. https://www.ncbi.nlm.nih.gov/pmc/articles/PMC3556554/

Chapter 16. Sacral Neuromodulation for Vulvodynia

[1]. Elneil, S. (2012). "Fact Sheet: Sacral Neuromodulation in Pelvic Floor Disorders Therapy Helps Normalize Organ Function." International Modulation Society. https://www.neuromodulation.com/assets/documents/Fact_Sheets/fact_sheet_ pelvic_floor_disorders.pdf

[2]. Roy H, Offiah I, Dua A. (2018). "Neuromodulation for Pelvic and Urogenital Pain." Brain Science, 2018 Oct; 8(10): 180. https://www.ncbi.nlm.nih.gov/pmc/articles/PMC6209873/

[3]. Ramsay, L. B., et al. (2009). "Sacral neuromodulation in the treatment of vulvar vestibulitis syndrome." Obstetrics and Gynecology, 114(2 PART 2 SUPPL.), 487-489. https://experts.umn.edu/en/publications/sacral-neuromodulation-in-the-treatment-of-vulvar-vestibulitis-sy

Chapter 17. Foods and Supplements for Vulvodynia

[1]. Joseph Bennington-Castro (2018). "How Your Diet and Other Factors Can Cause or Prevent Yeast Infections." Everyday Health. https://www.everydayhealth.com/yeast-infection/guide/prevention/

[2]. Caroline Knight (2020). "Can Food Allergies Cause Vulvodynia?" Vuvatech. https://www.vuvatech.com/blogs/care/can-food-allergies-cause-vulvodynia

[3]. Celiac.com (2007). "Vulvodynia And Celiac Disease." https://www.celiac.com/forums/topic/34421-vulvodynia-and-celiac-disease/

[4]. Drummond J, Ford D, Daniel S, Meyerink T. "Vulvodynia and Irritable Bowel Syndrome Treated With an Elimination Diet: A Case Report." Integrative Medicine (Encinitas, Calif.). 2016 Aug; 15(4):42-47. https://europepmc.org/article/pmc/4991650

[5]. National Center for Complementary and Integrative Health (2020). "Probiotics: What You Need to Know." https://nccih.nih.gov/health/probiotics/introduction.htm

[6]. Vulval Pain Society (2019). "The low-oxalate diet." http://www.vulvalpainsociety.org/vps/index.php/treatments/the-low-oxalate-diet

[7]. Harlow BL, Abenhaim HA, Vitonis AF, Harnack L. "Influence of dietary oxalates on the risk of adult-onset vulvodynia." The Journal of Reproductive Medicine. 2008 Mar; 53(3):171-178. https://europepmc.org/article/med/18441720

[8]. Drummond, Jessica (2018). "Functional Nutrition Treatment of Vulvodynia, Irritable Bowel Syndrome, and Depression: A Case Report." Integrative Med (Encinitas). 2018 Jun; 17(3): 44–51. https://www.ncbi.nlm.nih.gov/pmc/articles/PMC6396768/

[9]. Drummond, Jessica (2018). "Using an Elimination Diet to Relieve Vulvodynia and IBS." The Integrative Women's Health Institute. https://integrativewomenshealthinstitute.com/using-elimination-diet-relieve-vulvodynia-ibs/

Chapter 18. Acupuncture, Vaginal Acupressure, and Manual Trigger Point Therapy for Vulvodynia

[1]. Nagandla, G. & Sivalingam, N. (2014). "Vulvodynia: integrating current knowledge into clinical practice." Obstetrics & Gynaecology. https://obgyn.onlinelibrary.wiley.com/doi/full/10.1111/tog.12130

[2]. NIH (2019). "Effect of Two Acupuncture Protocols on Vulvodynia (Acu/Vulpain)." https://clinicaltrials.gov/ct2/show/NCT03481621

[3]. Schlaeger JM, Pauls HA, Powell-Roach KL, et al. Vulvodynia, "A Really Great Torturer": A Mixed Methods Pilot Study Examining Pain Experiences and Drug/Non-drug Pain Relief Strategies. J Sex Med 2019;16:1255–63. doi:10.1016/j.jsxm.2019.05.004

[4]. Schlaegar et al. (2015). "Acupuncture for the Treatment of Vulvodynia: A Randomized Wait-List Controlled Pilot Study." The Journal of Sexual Medicine 2015 Vol 12, Issue 4, April 2015. https://www.sciencedirect.com/science/article/pii/S1743609515309899

[5]. Vincent C. The safety of acupuncture. *BMJ* 2001;323:467–8. doi:10.1136/bmj.323.7311.467

[6]. Ventegodt et al (2006). "Clinical Holistic Medicine: Holistic Sexology and Acupressure Through the Vagina (Hippocratic Pelvic Massage)." Semantic Scholar. https://www.semanticscholar.org/paper/Clinical-Holistic-Medicine%3A-Holistic-Sexology-and-Ventegodt-Clausen/6bae97b7f3142ccd960caa06165ddab5638fe936

[7]. The American College of Obstetricians and Gynecologists (2017). "Glossary." https://www.acog.org/Patients/FAQs/Vulvodynia?IsMobileSet=false

Chapter 19. TENS for Vulvodynia

[1]. Vallinga et al. (2014). "Transcutaneous electrical nerve stimulation as an additional treatment for women suffering from therapy-resistant provoked vestibulodynia: a feasibility study." Journal of Sexual Medicine 2015 Jan;12(1):228-37, reported in NCBI. https://www.ncbi.nlm.nih.gov/pubmed/25388372

[2]. Medical News Today (2018). "What is a TENS unit and does it work?" https://www.medicalnewstoday.com/articles/323632

[3]. Smart Patients (2020). "Intra-vaginal Electrical Stimulation Device Compared to Sham Device for Chronic Pelvic Pain." https://www.smartpatients.com/trials/NCT02397785

[4]. Vance et al. "Using TENS for pain control: the state of the evidence". Pain Management. 2014 May; 4(3):197-209. https://www.ncbi.nlm.nih.gov/pmc/articles/PMC4186747/

[5]. Murina F, Felice R, Di Francesco S, Oneda S. Vaginal diazepam plus transcutaneous electrical nerve stimulation to treat vestibulodynia: A randomized controlled trial. Eur J Obstet Gynecol Reprod Biol. 2018 Sep; 228:148-153. https://pubmed.ncbi.nlm.nih.gov/29960200/

[6]. Electrotherpy. TheInternational Society for Electrophysical Agents in Physical Therapy (ISEAPT) (2020). "Transcutaneous Electrical Nerve Stimulation (TENS)." http://www.electrotherapy.org/modality/transcutaneous-electrical-nerve-stimulation-tens

Chapter 20. Yoga and Diaphragmatic Breathing for Vulvodynia

[1]. Wong, Cathy (2019). "How to Do Belly Breathing." Very Well Health. https://www.verywellhealth.com/how-to-breathe-with-your-belly-89853

[2]. Howard, Leslie (N.d.). "Core Connection: The Relationship Between the Pelvic Floor & the Breath." Yoga U. https://www.yogauonline.com/contributor-posts/core-connection-relationship-between-pelvic-floor-breath

[3]. Your Pace Yoga (N.d.). "Yoga for Vulvodynia." https://yourpaceyoga.com/blog/yoga-for-vulvodynia/

[4]. Maidansky, Rebecca (2018). "3 Exercises That Can Make Sex Less Painful, According to a Pelvic Floor Therapist." Health.com https://www.health.com/sexual-health/pelvic-floor-exercises-painful-sex

Chapter 21. Psychological Treatment for Vulvodynia

[1]. Nagandla, G. & Sivalingam, N. (2014). "Vulvodynia: integrating current knowledge into clinical practice." Obstetrics & Gynaecology. https://obgyn.onlinelibrary.wiley.com/doi/full/10.1111/tog.12130

[2]. Dunkley, C.R; Brotto, L.A. (2016). Psychological Treatments for Provoked Vestibulodynia: Integration of Mindfulness-Based and Cognitive Behavioral Therapies. Journal of Clinical Psychology. https://www.researchgate.net/publication/299475036_Psychological_Treatments_for_Provoked_Vestibulodynia_Integration_of_Mindfulness-Based_and_Cognitive_Behavioral_Therapies/link/5ccb0a2e92851c3c2f81677f/download

[3]. Shiel, W.C. (2018). "Medical Definition of Randomized Controlled Trial." Medicinenet. https://www.medicinenet.com/script/main/art.asp?articlekey=39532

[4]. Comprehensive Meta-Analysis (2019). "Why perform a meta-analysis?" https://www.meta-analysis.com/pages/why_do.php?cart=

[5]. Science Direct (2019). "Allostatic Load." https://www.sciencedirect.com/topics/neuroscience/allostatic-load

[6]. Henzell et al. (2017). "Provoked vestibulodynia: current perspectives." International Journal of Women's Health. https://jeanhailes.org.au/contents/documents/Health_Professionals/Webinars/IJWH-provoked-vestibulodynia--current-perspectives_091117.pdf

Chapter 22. Surgical Intervention for Vulvodynia

[1]. The Vulva Pain Society (2019). "Published Research."
http://www.vulvalpainsociety.org/vps/index.php/research/published-
research#Vestibulectomystudy

[2]. The Vulva Pain Society (2019). "Surgery for Vulva Pain."
http://www.vulvalpainsociety.org/vps/index.php/treatments/surgery-for-vulval-
pain

[3]. Traas MA, Bekkers RL, Dony JM, et al. (2006). "Surgical treatment for the vulvar
vestibulitis syndrome." Obstet Gynecol. 2006;107(2 Pt 1):256-262.
https://pubmed.ncbi.nlm.nih.gov/16449109/

[4]. Eva LJ, et al. (2008). "Is Modified Vestibulectomy for Localized Provoked
Vulvodynia an Effective Long-Term Treatment? A Follow-Up Study."
J Reprod Med.2008 Jun;53(6):435-40.
https://pubmed.ncbi.nlm.nih.gov/18664062/

[5]. Tommola, P. et al. (2006). "Surgical treatment of vulvar vestibulitis: a review."
Obstetrics & Gynecology: February 2006 - Volume 107 - Issue 2 - p 256-262
https://journals.lww.com/greenjournal/fulltext/2006/02000/surgical_treatme
nt_for_the_vulvar_vestibulitis.9.aspx_

Living with Vulvodynia

Chapter 23. Relationships and Living with Vulvodynia

[1]. National Vulvodynia Association (2016). "My Partner Has Vulvodynia – What Do I
Need to Know? A Self-Help Guide for Partners." www.nva.org

[2]. Nguyen et al. "Comfort in discussing vulvar pain in social relationships among
women with vulvodynia". *J Reprod Med*. 2012 Mar-Apr;57(3-4):109-14.

Chapter 24. Sexual Intimacy and Vulvodynia

[1]. Fetters, A. (2019). "What Happens to Relationships When Sex Hurts."
https://www.theatlantic.com/family/archive/2019/11/vulvodynia-painful-sex-
women/601567/

[2]. National Vulvodynia Association (2021). "Overcoming Challenges in Your
Intimate Relationship." https://www.nva.org/learnpatient/overcoming-
challenges-in-your-intimate-
relationship/#:~:text=Chronic%20pain%2C%20and%20especially%20vulvodyni
a,of%20desire%20in%20either%20partner

[3]. Kelly, J. (2019). "Living with vulvodynia: can I enjoy a healthy sex life?" The
Femedic.

Chapter 25. Pregnancy and Giving Birth for Vulvodynia Patients

[1]. Johnson et al. (2015). "You have to go through it and have your children: reproductive experiences among women with vulvodynia." BMC Pregnancy and Childbirth. 2015; 15: 114.
https://www.ncbi.nlm.nih.gov/pmc/articles/PMC4518563/

[2]. The Vulva Pain Society (2020). "Pregnancy and vulval pain."
http://www.vulvalpainsociety.org/vps/index.php/advice-and-self-help/pregnancy

[3]. Nguyen et al. (2012). "A Population-Based Study of Pregnancy and Delivery Characteristics Among Women with Vulvodynia." Pain Therapy. 2012 Dec; 1(1): 2. https://www.ncbi.nlm.nih.gov/pmc/articles/PMC4107863/

[4]. The American Pain Society (N.d.). "The Journal of Pain."
https://www.jpain.org/article/S1526-5900(14)00168-0/pdf

[5]. Fontaine, Melinda (2016). "Pregnancy, Labor, and Delivery with Vulvovaginal Pain." https://pelvicpainrehab.com/female-pelvic-pain/4010/pregnancy-labor-delivery-vulvovaginal-pain/

[6]. Shah, S., Banh, E. T., Koury, K., Bhatia, G., Nandi, R., & Gulur, P. (2015). "Pain Management in Pregnancy: Multimodal Approaches." *Pain research and treatment*, 2015, 987483. https://doi.org/10.1155/2015/987483

Chapter 26. Evidence-Based Medicine

[1]. "This Girl is on Fire. Sensemaking in an Online Health Community for Vulvodynia." Conference Paper 2019.
https://dl.acm.org/doi/10.1145/3290605.3300359 and
https://www.researchgate.net/publication/332747590_This_Girl_is_on_Fire_S ensemaking_in_an_Online_Health_Community_for_Vulvodynia

Chapter 27. Ongoing Research Trials for Vulvodynia

[1]. https://www.nva.org/research/

[2]. Clinical Trials (2020). https://www.clinicaltrials.gov/

Chapter 28. Patient Stories

[1]. National Vulvodynia Association (2019). "Patient Stories."
https://www.nva.org/for-patients/patient-stories/

[2]. The London Pain Clinic (2020). "Patient Stories."

Chapter 29. Organizations, Support Groups, and Online Health Communities (OHC) for Women with Vulvodynia and Vulvar Pain

[1]. Peers for Progress (2021). "Science Behind Peer Support." http://peersforprogress.org/learn-about-peer-support/science-behind-peer-support/

Chapter 30. Claiming Disability Benefit

[1]. National Vulvodynia Association (2019). "How to Apply for Disability Benefits: A Self-Help Guide for Women with Vulvodynia." https://www.nva.org/

[2]. Gov.UK (2020). "Financial Help If You're Disabled." https://www.gov.uk/financial-help-disabled/disability-and-sickness-benefits

Chapter 31. Basic Gynecological Terminology

[1]. Medical News Today (2017). "How does acupuncture work?" https://www.medicalnewstoday.com/articles/156488.php

[2]. The American College of Obstetricians and Gynecologists (2017). "Glossary." https://www.acog.org/Patients/FAQs/Vulvodynia?IsMobileSet=false

[3]. Mandal, Ananya (2019. "What are Cannabinoids?" https://www.news-medical.net/health/What-are-Cannabinoids.aspx

[4]. The Centers for Vulvovagina Disorders (2020). "Clitoral Pain." http://vulvodynia.com/conditions/clitoral-pain

[5]. Mayo Clinic (2018). "Painful intercourse (dyspareunia)." https://www.mayoclinic.org/diseases-conditions/painful-intercourse/symptoms-causes/syc-20375967

[6]. Andrews, Jeffrey Campbell (2010). "Vulvodynia: An Evidence-Based Approach to Medical Management." JCOM journal Vol. 17, No. 5 May 2010. https://www.nva.org/wp-content/uploads/2016/03/Vulvodynia-an-evidence-based-approach-to-medical-management.pdf

[7]. Healthline (2017). "What is nociceptive pain?" https://www.healthline.com/health/nociceptive-pain

[8]. International Society for Sexual Medicine (2020). "What is provoked vestibulodynia (PVD)?" https://www.issm.info/sexual-health-qa/what-is-provoked-vestibulodynia-pvd/

Appendix A. Popular Oral Medications Which Can be Prescribed for Vulvodynia

[1]. Drugs (2019). Medications for Vulvodynia.
https://www.drugs.com/condition/vulvodynia.html

[2]. Andrews, Jeffrey Campbell (2010). Vulvodynia: An Evidence-Based Approach to Medical Management. Journal of Clinical Outcomes Management. Vol. 17, No. 5 May 2010. https://www.nva.org/wp-content/uploads/2016/03/Vulvodynia-an-evidence-based-approach-to-medical-management.pdf

[3]. Loflin B.J, Westmoreland K, Williams NT (2019). Vulvodynia: A Review of the Literature. J Pharm Technol. 2019;35(1):11–24.
https://www.ncbi.nlm.nih.gov/pmc/articles/PMC6313270/#!po=22.8261

[4]. NHS (2019). Dosulepin. https://www.nhs.uk/medicines/dosulepin/

[5]. Psycom (2019). Uses of Lamictal (Lamotrigine) as a Mood Stabilizer.
https://www.psycom.net/depression.central.lamotrigine.html

[6]. National Institute for Health and Care Excellence (2020). BNF Antidepressant drugs. [Online] Available at: https://bnf.nice.org.uk/treatment-summary/antidepressant-drugs.html [Accessed 22 June 2020]

[7]. National Institute for Health and Care Excellence (2020). Amitriptyline Hydrochloride. [Online] Available at:
https://bnf.nice.org.uk/drug/amitriptyline-hydrochloride.html [Accessed 22 June 2020]

[8]. National Institute for Health and Care Excellence (2020). Paroxetine. [Online] Available at: https://bnf.nice.org.uk/drug/paroxetine.html [Accessed 22 June 2020]

[9]. National Institute for Health and Care Excellence (2020). Duloxetine. [Online] Available at: https://bnf.nice.org.uk/drug/duloxetine.html#indicationsAndDoses [Accessed 22 June 2020]

[10]. National Vulvodynia Association (2020). Vulvodynia treatments. [Online] Available at: https://www.nva.org/learnpatient/medical-management/ [Accessed 22 June 2020]

[11]. Faye. R.B. and Piraccini. E. (2020) Vulodynia. StatPearls, [Online]. Available at: https://www.ncbi.nlm.nih.gov/books/NBK430792/ [Accessed 22 June 2020]

[12]. National Institute for Health and Care Excellence (2020). Topiramate. [Online] Available at:
https://bnf.nice.org.uk/drug/topiramate.html#indicationsAndDoses [Accessed 22 June 2020]

[13]. National Institute for Health and Care Excellence (2020). Benzodiazepines. [Online] Available at: https://bnf.nice.org.uk/drug-class/benzodiazepines.html [Accessed 22 June 2020]

[14]. Drugs (2019). "Medications for Vulvodynia."
https://www.drugs.com/condition/vulvodynia.html

[15]. Andrews, Jeffrey Campbell (2010). "Vulvodynia: An Evidence-Based Approach to Medical Management." Journal of Clinical Outcomes Management. Vol. 17, No. 5

May 2010. https://www.nva.org/wp-content/uploads/2016/03/Vulvodynia-an-evidence-based-approach-to-medical-management.pdf

[16]. Loflin BJ, Westmoreland K, Williams NT (2019). "Vulvodynia: A Review of the Literature." J Pharm Technol. 2019;35(1):11–24.
https://www.ncbi.nlm.nih.gov/pmc/articles/PMC6313270/#!po=22.8261

[17]. NHS (2019). "Dosulepin." https://www.nhs.uk/medicines/dosulepin/

[18]. Psycom (2019). "Uses of Lamictal (Lamotrigine) as a Mood Stabilizer."
https://www.psycom.net/depression.central.lamotrigine.html

CPSIA information can be obtained
at www.ICGtesting.com
Printed in the USA
BVHW051642130723
667200BV00006B/146